The
DEVIL'S
INTERVENTION
into
Healthcare
Politics
Churches
Courts
Families

Dr. Chester A. Wilk

- **How to prevent divorces and save marriages**
- **How to cure our "sick" healthcare system**
- **How to beat the devil at his own game**
- **How to maximize your healthcare**
- **The devil proven more than a symbol of evil**

Copyright

The Devil's Intervention into Healthcare Politics,
Churches, Courts, Families

Copyright © 2013 by Chester A. Wilk, D.C.

First Edition © 2013

ISBN 978-1-4675-5727-6

Printed in the United States of America.

Author
Chester A. Wilk, D.C.
P.O. Box 81
Park Ridge, IL 60068

web: www.chetwilk.com   or   www.chesterwilk.com

Edited by C.L. Stewart,
http://www.writereditorforyou.com

Dedication

I dedicate this book to my wife, Ardith, and to my daughters, Kim, Cathy, and Cindy.

Contents

Chapter 1

The Devil Gets into Healthcare

The devil has been very active in healthcare, while most people do not even realize or recognize that the devil plays a major role in it. How can the devil cause the most divisiveness, polarization, pain, suffering, and death with human ailments? The answer is to get into a key position within a medical organization, like the American Medical Association, disseminate his lies, and create all kinds of problems in healthcare.

Let's look at the facts.

The AMA formed a committee on quackery, which sounded noble on the surface, as though they were going to clean up their own profession from dishonest medical doctors. However, this committee was NOT concerned with cleaning up its own house, but with eliminating chiropractic care. The devil is a skillful divider, persecutor, imposter, impersonator, and hypocrite, so you can see how he manipulated the committee. The strategy was to create a lie about a group of people and then eliminate them.

The architect of the AMA quackery committee was a lawyer by the name of Doyl Taylor. He was not only the secretary of this infamous AMA quackery committee, but also the chairman of the AMA Department of Investigation, which made him the most powerful and influential employee of the AMA.

He couldn't be put into a more perfect position by Satan to create division and mayhem within the healthcare industry.

Doyl Taylor was both arrogant and foolish enough to put his intent in writing, to work covertly behind the scene, create a lie about the chiropractic profession, and then try to eliminate it altogether. Once he could create a lie about chiropractic care being an unscientific cult, he could forbid medical doctors from associating with chiropractors by labeling it "unethical." Therefore, any medical doctor choosing to associate with a chiropractor could be called before his committee and be punished for doing so.

During this time, it was a fact that 3,000 people were dying every week from unnecessary surgeries and prescription medications! Nobody questioned the accuracy of these statistics. The medical journals openly admitted to them. What is worse is that these unnecessary deaths have increased every year.

The AMA wanted to make matters even worse by dividing our healthcare system and eliminating chiropractors that could make major contributions to reducing these deaths.

In their attempt to malign chiropractic care, the AMA propaganda relied on using innuendoes, information taken out of context, half-truths, obsolete information, obscure information sources, exceptional cases, and outright false statements.

This is the way the devil works. He will take some truth and mix it in with lies, or take information out of context and use it to defame an entire profession.

The main theme of the AMA's propaganda campaign was that chiropractic care was a worthless, dangerous, and unscientific cult. Nothing could be further from the truth.

2

Regarding Being Unscientific.

Science can be described as systematized knowledge derived from observation, study, and experimentation conducted in order to determine the nature of the thing being studied.

With respect to chiropractic, researchers have applied specific types of treatments, called adjustments, to groups of people with certain ailments, and, through carefully-controlled studies, have been able to achieve consistent and predictable results, and to have both doctors (objectively) and patients (subjectively) agree that the chiropractic treatments affected the desired improvement. This completely fulfills the requirements of being a scientifically based profession.

Chiropractic's Clinical and Therapeutic Effectiveness.

The world-renowned RAND Corporation *(The acronym stands for research and development.)* is the largest "think tank" in the United States, outside of a university.

RAND found that there is **more randomized controlled studies proving the effectiveness of chiropractic care than there are for many of the therapies presently being used by medical doctors.**

There are also government and hospital studies from the United States, Canada, Great Britain, New Zealand, and Italy, proving chiropractic's safety and therapeutic effectiveness.

A study conducted by AVMED, which was the largest Health Maintenance Organization (HMO) in the Southeastern United States, showed chiropractic to be both clinically and scientifically-based, safer, and often **therapeutically superior** to a medical-surgical approach to healthcare.

The Safety of Chiropractic.

Actuarial studies performed for insurance carriers are by far the most reliable indicators of the safety of a profession, because there is no room for emotion or bias within actuarial studies, as they are used to determine how much of an insurance premium a doctor must pay to practice in their profession.

Insurance carriers who insure doctors based on the safety of their profession have ranked chiropractic care as being the safest healthcare profession in the world. There is none safer.

A chiropractor can purchase an entire year of malpractice insurance for about the same price as some medical physicians and surgeons pay to purchase just one week of malpractice coverage! This speaks for itself.

The safety of chiropractic care is superabundantly proven to be extremely safe, while medicine is ranked by actuaries as one of the most dangerous.

The Dishonesty and Hypocrisy of the AMA.

The disingenuous attitude of the AMA can be illustrated by its own actions. It had a clinical outcome study done on chiropractic within a military hospital during WWII, led by Dr. Irvin Hendryson, who was a member of the AMA board of trustees.

The military hospital study showed that chiropractic care was very effective, but the AMA suppressed this information for over 60 years until, under our subpoena, the AMA was forced to grudgingly release this study to avoid facing a contempt of court citation. The study also found that pregnant women under chiropractic care had an easier time in delivering children. Hence, the AMA disseminated information that totally contra-indicated its own clinical findings, which was patently dishonest.

An Informant from the AMA Steps Forward.

The AMA's secret committee memos were made public by an informant within the AMA, which revealed "The <u>primary mission</u> of the AMA Committee on Quackery was first the containment, and then the ultimate elimination, of chiropractic care." The author of this written memo was both arrogant and stupid enough to put his entire plan in writing, which was an open admission of committing antitrust.

The infamous AMA committee wrote that they intended to get the chiropractic colleges to **"wither on the vine and die an undramatic death!"** Their strategy was to destroy the image of chiropractic healthcare so badly that colleges would not get new applicants and ultimately would have to close their doors.

Dr. Jerome McAndrews, who was President of the Palmer College of Chiropractic, and later Executive Director of the International Chiropractors Association, very appropriately referred to the AMA as an "evil empire."

I view the nebulous function of the AMA committee to be on the same level of dangerous deceit and quackery as the *"Showers of Auschwitz."*

Only the devil could get an organization like the AMA to resort to such ugly tactics.

My battle was not with the AMA as such, but with the devil who was able to insert himself into the minds and hearts of key individuals and cause such harm.

An Antitrust Lawsuit Had to Be Filed.

The malicious lies, as well as the antitrust conduct of the American Medical Association Quackery Committee was so outrageous and illegal that the AMA had to be taken to court, and I believe the devil was behind it!

Healthy competition forces businesses to provide the best products and services they can deliver, at the best possible prices. Let's suppose Chrysler, Ford, or General Motors formed a committee with a noble-sounding name like *"Committee on Automotive Quality,"* whose primary mission, *boldly stated in writing,* was to contain and eliminate its competition by slandering them so that consumer confidence and car sales would drop, and they were forced out of business.

If this happened, you would see the biggest antitrust lawsuit in history, which would ruin the guilty automaker.

This is precisely what the AMA tried to do with chiropractic.

When Taylor became a named defendant in our lawsuit and was summoned to go to court to testify, he fled to Arizona, which was out of the jurisdiction of the Northern Illinois Federal Court. He ran like a coward and had his son come to court and say that his dad had crippling arthritis and could not appear in court to testify. We were able to prove that Taylor was actually on the golf course every day, playing golf, which is hardly a pastime for someone claiming to be too crippled to show up in a courtroom to testify.

A video deposition was eventually taken of Taylor while he was in Arizona, and he admitted under oath that he did not know if his propaganda was truthful or dishonest—***and he didn't care!***

He spent 11 years and millions of dollars working covertly behind the scenes to create a false image of chiropractic care—as people were dying every day, unnecessarily.

I even went to the Justice Department and urged them to file an amicus brief and come in as a friend of the court, yet they refused to act. The devil was so firmly entrenched within our government that both the Justice Department and the Federal Trade Commission (FTC) failed to do their jobs.

This is what the United States Department of Justice and the Federal Trade Commission (FTC) are supposed to do—protect the chiropractic profession from illegal antitrust conduct against it.

The way the lawsuit got started was when an informant from the AMA smuggled out internal secret documents revealing the AMA's plan to eliminate chiropractic and published these documents into a book.

The informant drove to the Palmer College of Chiropractic and dropped off a truckload of books, received nominal payment for them, gave the college permission to make duplicate copies, and then disappeared. The original books had a Nazi swastika superimposed over the AMA emblem because of the similar propaganda tactics used by the AMA against chiropractors.

When the college made reprints, they removed the Nazi swastika from the cover. The informant was given the name of "Sore Throat," after "Deep Throat," taken from the Watergate scandal. After *"In the Public Interest"* came out, I was contacted by Attorney Jerry Hosier, who had received a copy of the book from his close friend. Mr. Hosier said if the documents in the book were legitimate, then chiropractors had a per se violation of the antitrust laws.

Dr. Jerome McAndrews, Executive Director of the ICA, had a brother named George, who was a lawyer. George McAndrews was called in to find a qualified law firm that had antitrust experience to handle the case. Numerous law firms were contacted, but they either had a conflict of interest about representing drug companies or they were too small to handle a lawsuit of this size.

Having come from a family of 25 chiropractors, including his own father, brother, and sister, George McAndrews realized that he could not turn his back on the chiropractic healthcare profession by refusing to take the case.

The antitrust lawsuit was actually filed against 14 individuals and organizations, although the AMA was the primary defendant. We were literally taking on the entire medical establishment.

The defendants all settled, but it came down to the principle defendant, which was the AMA. The lawsuit took 14 years and had to go to the Supreme Court twice before we chiropractors eventually won the case.

The AMA reportedly spent 20 million dollars and lost. The AMA had to publish a statement in their journal admitting their wrongdoings and that it was all right for medical physicians to associate professionally with chiropractors. What happened during this 14-year battle would make an incredible motion picture. It has the plot, intrigue, conspiracy, covert activity, shameless conduct, and dishonesty that would be more dramatic than the best John Grisham novel—especially because it is a true story.

I believe that one day an enterprising motion picture producer will see the sensational story and make a motion picture out of our amazing court case. The real hero in this drama was Attorney George McAndrews, because of his incredible knowledge, courage, commitment, and tenacity.

I was convinced that God played a major role in what was happening, which was to bring closer inter-professional cooperation between all healthcare professions and save thousands of human lives in the process.

On the Side of the Angels.

When Attorney McAndrews went to the AMA headquarters, the AMA counsel told him that they had a $40-million-dollar-a-year budget, that they would drag his case on forever, and that he could never win. George responded by looking the counselor straight in the face and telling him that he would one day float the Battleship

8

Missouri down the Saint Lawrence Seaway and park it at Navy Pier for the unconditional surrender of the AMA—and added that when he did this, they should all wear top hats. He likened it to the unconditional surrender of the Japanese at the end of WWII. *(Can you imagine seeing this in a motion picture?)*

George never seemed to be down, and was always finding humor in whatever he was doing. When he was in the courtroom one day, surrounded by 25 lawyers, one of them said, *"Hey George, where's your assistant?"*

These were the leading counsels from the biggest law firms in the country. However, I believe that the Good Lord was on George's side, which made him the majority in the courtroom.

George responded, "When I get busy, I'll get one. But, in the meantime, I'll just step into the phone booth and disrobe!"

Using Superman's tactics as a source humor was a great way for George to maintain his sanity in the very stressful situation in which he found himself.

One of the lawyers who worked with Attorney McAndrews said that it was hard to get emotional about a typical antitrust case, since he would normally see one wealthy major corporation fighting another major wealthy corporation over selfish interests, but in our case, he felt like he was on the side of the angels.

It took divine guidance from God to put George in the exact time and place to do what no man in the entire world *could have—or would have—done!* This was actually a greater accomplishment than David's triumph over Goliath. All David had to do was place a stone between the eyes of Goliath.

George had to take on a *dozen opponents all at one time,* and ultimately prevail in the battle. George was given extraordinary talent, which had to come from God.

9

Amazingly, George graduated from Notre Dame University with the highest grade-point average ever attained by anyone in the history of the school! Of the millions of graduates, for him to be #1 was not mere coincidence. This was Divine Intervention.

When George took the American Bar examination, he scored the highest grade ever attained by anyone from the State of Illinois.

All of George's amazing talent wasn't coincidental. He was chosen by God to perform what no other lawyer *could or would* have done. He is a true servant of God and he did what he had to do valiantly.

Today, we find medical doctors contacting chiropractors with letters, offering to cooperate with them on cases that may need medical or surgical attention, which was something that would not have happened before the lawsuit, and it came about thanks to Attorney George McAndrews. It was a step in the right direction.

A Modern Day Medical Holocaust.

Suppose there was an organized terrorist group of individuals in America who openly took credit for killing 100 people every week. How would the public react? We would see a major public outcry and a demand that appropriate action be taken immediately to stop this senseless killing and suffering.

Suppose there was a group that took credit for killing 3,000, or 30 times more deaths a week. How do you suppose the public would react?

Amazing as it sounds, there is such a group, and it is called the medical profession, which actually admits to causing 3,000 deaths a week and 150,000 deaths a year from unnecessary drugs and surgery. They admit to it in their own journals! Add hospital errors to these statistics and the total increases to 783,936 unnecessary deaths a year.

Recently, researchers Gary Null, Ph.D., Carolyn Dean, M.D., N.D., Martin Feldman, M.D., Debora Rasio, M.D., and Dorothy Smith, Ph.D. authored a paper titled "Death by Medicine" that presents strong evidence about today's healthcare system and how it has not improved, but has become even worse.

Their report states, *"It is now evident that the American medical system is the leading cause of death and injury in the US."*

Here are some of their findings:

- The number of unnecessary medical and surgical procedures performed annually is 7.5 million per year.

- The number of people having in-hospital, adverse reactions to prescribed drugs was found to be 2.2 million per year.

- The number of unnecessary antibiotics prescribed annually for viral infections is 20 million per year.

- The number of people exposed to unnecessary hospitalization annually is 8.9 million per year.

And, the most shocking statistic of all...

- The total number of deaths caused by conventional medicine is an astounding 783,936 per year.

Even though additional healthcare statistics just as shocking as those mentioned above can be found in numerous medical journals, little or nothing is being done to correct this appalling situation.

Why is there no outcry?

I believe that the devil has been able to blindfold an entire nation into ignoring it. One of the devil's tools is greed and the unholy economic alliance between the drug houses and the MD's

Some of the Dire Consequences of Abusive and Excessive Over-Utilization of Drugs and Surgery.

1. MD's are now the leading cause of death and injury in America.

2. Prescription drugs kill more people than traffic accidents, guns, AIDS, breast cancer, diabetes, respiratory diseases, and stroke.

3. Every 14 minutes, someone dies from prescription medications.

4. MD's went on strike in Los Angeles County in 1979; the death rate dropped by 153 people since elective surgery was not being performed.

5. The World Health Organization (WHO) states that the United States is rated #1, meaning it is the most expensive healthcare in the world, yet we ranked #37 in the world for quality of care.

6. Our healthcare system has created drug addicts of epidemic proportions. In 2010, an estimated 20.1 million or 8 percent of our population are addicted to drugs! (Source: *Substance Abuse and Mental Health Services Administration of the U.S. Dept. of Health and Human Services*)

7. Medical expenses cause 62 percent of all bankruptcies in America—more than all the other reasons combined. Seventy-five percent were people who had health insurance.

   This puts the average family in America one major hospitalization away from bankruptcy.

8. Our healthcare system is a misnomer; it is "disease care" that is costly, inefficient, and dangerous. The proverbial ounce of prevention is ignored. Instead of encouraging healthy lifestyles, the drug companies tell people to take pills for whatever ails them.

9. More people die from prescription drugs than from heroin and cocaine combined. (Source: *Centers for Disease Control and Prevention.*) The CDC study found that enough drugs are prescribed annually to medicate every adult in America every day for a month.

10. Patients with viral conditions have been given antibiotic drugs, which are proven to be inappropriate and ineffective on viruses, causing the bacteria to mutate and become more resistant to the antibiotic drugs—the bacteria are winning the battle.

11. Examples of the Excessive Markup on Drugs:

Prozac: 20 mg. tablets cost $247.47, ingredients cost 11 cents = **224,973 percent mark-up!**

Xanax: 100 tablets cost $136.79, ingredients cost 2.4 cents = **569,958 percent mark-up!**

Celebrex: 100 tablets cost $130.27, ingredients cost 60 cents = **21,712 percent mark-up!**

In addition to being expensive, Prozac is no more effective than taking sugar pills, while its negative effects on children, by upsetting the production of neuro-transmitters, can cause violent behavior and even suicide.

The end result of this greed and lack of quality care is <u>thousands of unnecessary deaths</u> every week, needless suffering, iatrogenic drug reactions, medical malpractice lawsuits, and an overly expensive, polarized, and destructive healthcare system, which needs serious reform. Not even the U.S. government can afford it.

Chiropractic, which focuses on facilitating the body's natural God-given healing capacity, was once unsuccessfully targeted for extermination by the AMA using Nazi tactics! *(e.g. create a lie about a profession and try to eliminate it).* **The U.S. Federal Court found the AMA guilty of antitrust.**

Medicine cannot effectively correct all health care

problems by itself. This is where chiropractic needs to work closer in all of our general hospitals in America, utilizing its unique and special services where it is shown to be superior, safer, and more cost-effective.

Today, **an unholy alliance exists between the drug companies and MD's** that put profits above what is in the best interest of patients. Chiropractic, which is often ignored, can provide better and safer methods of health care without deadly side effects.

The reason our nation is not outraged by the 3,000 medical/surgical deaths every week is because the pharmaceutical industry and the devil have ***de-sensitized the American population to the grave seriousness of how they are causing unnecessary deaths!***

The next time you watch television, take note of the many repetitious television ads that are played that promote toxic drugs every 8 to 10 minutes during your favorite TV program. We, as a nation, have become so de-sensitized to these ads that even though the law forces the drug companies to list the dangerous and often deadly consequences caused by each drug, we no longer hear the truth. We even go so far as to follow the ad's advice to "Ask your doctor if XZY is right for you."

We are witnessing ***a modern day medical holocaust***. This may sound like an extreme statement to make, but the statistics clearly prove my point.

Any proposed health care insurance plan relating to our existing health care system would be like putting a band-aid over a hemorrhage. Our healthcare system is sick and it needs to be reformed before it can be effectively insured.

Avandia was FDA approved, despite an estimated 83,000 deaths caused by this drug, while the lawyers sat perched like a bunch of vultures ready to capitalize on it. Its side effects include heart attack, congestive heart failure, stroke, liver failure, bone fracture, and death. This toxic drug is also still on the market.

It is almost like a conspiracy between lawyers and the FDA. There isn't any wonder why malpractice insurance for MDs is going through the roof.

We could fill volumes of books about such drug reactions, and these examples are not even the tip of the iceberg.

This is NOT intended to discourage or malign good medicine, but to inform people that although prescription medications can save lives, they can also take lives, so **intelligent and informed consumer utilization is critical**.

The obvious motive behind all of these drug advertisements is to make money for the drug houses. Healthcare consumers need to be made aware of the medical bias, which is not in their best interests.

Approximately 18 billion dollars is spent annually by drug companies to market their drugs to physicians. That's 1.5 billion dollars a month!

Tens of thousands of drug sales representatives converge on medical physicians <u>every day</u> trying to sell them on their drugs.

Most physicians do not realize that the pharmaceutical houses spend **$10,000 per doctor every year,** with perks and gifts to influence their thinking.

Deaths from all major airline crashes in the U.S. amount to less than 300 annually, but one airline crash gets more **media attention and government scrutiny** than the 300 medication-related deaths that have been occurring **every day for decades**!

Deaths from drug-related reactions rarely look any different than natural deaths. The victims die quietly and un-dramatically in hospitals. There is no visual wreckage to videotape and no crash sites to fascinate and horrify television viewers. And as the media people say, "No film, no story."

The reported adverse effects of medications are only the tip of the iceberg. Consider **Digoxin** (also known as digitalis), a best-selling heart drug.

According to an article in *JAMA*, the Food and Drug Administration (FDA) received only 82 reports each year involving Digoxin, while Medicare records reveal 202,211 hospitalizations for Digoxin's adverse effects in a 7-year period. That comes to 28,000 reactions per year, while the FDA claims to have only heard about 82 of them.

Allergies to drugs are increasing to epidemic levels that would soon exceed bacterial diseases in number. Most medical experts agree that far too many drugs are being consumed. Forty-six percent of Americans take at least one prescription drug daily, while most of them are not necessary, according to medical experts.

Some conscientious medical physicians have criticized the drug industry, with its intense, diverse, and unrelenting efforts to influence physicians to sell more drugs, and are now calling for serious reform. The healthcare system is like an albatross around our nation's neck, because of the unholy alliance between the drug industry and medical physicians. It is a major factor causing our healthcare costs to go up and creating an economic crisis. Instead of healthcare being our friend, it has become our adversary.

How to Maximize Your Healthcare.

Many people are so heavily programmed to take prescription medications for every kind of symptom that they don't have a remote clue as to what constitutes a rational, safe, and effective approach to healthcare.

What you are about to read—and if you understand and practice this approach in your choice of healthcare—may be the most important thing for you to remember about treating ailments. It could even save your life!

If you follow these rules, you will be in at least the upper one or two-percent bracket of properly enlightened healthcare consumers.

First of all, to understand what represents rational, safe, and effective healthcare, we need to realize that appropriate healthcare falls into four different categories. These categories may be compared to *a four-legged stool*.

If you remove any one of these legs *(or healthcare approaches)*, the stool becomes unstable and cannot function effectively.

The four-legged stool is like the four different treatment categories or approaches to treating ailments. These are:

- The (Appropriate) Surgical Approach

- The Psychological Approach (which includes ministers, priests, and rabbis)

- The Chemical or Medical Approach

- The Structural/Biomechanical/Manipulative/ Adjustment Approach

We will examine each one individually. The object is to use the safest, least invasive, and most effective treatment first.

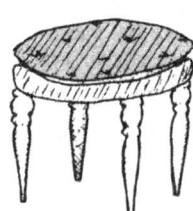

The (Appropriate) Surgical Approach.

If a person has appendicitis, a hernia, fracture, malignant tumor, herniated disc, a need for a hip or knee replacement, or any kind of muscular or structural deformity that hampers their normal ability to function, then surgical intervention more than likely is indicated.

Surgeons play an extremely vital and essential role in healthcare, but like any healthcare profession, surgical intervention needs to be used with respect to the safety and effectiveness of the treatment, and using the most conservative treatment first.

In 2010, a study reported in *The Journal of the American Medical Association (JAMA)* indicated that unnecessary surgeries are on the rise. Too many back surgeries are being performed and people are suffering as a result. JAMA wrote that doctors kill more people than auto accidents and guns combined.

There are 1.2 million spinal surgeries performed in the U.S. each year, and the number of surgeries keeps increasing. Recent studies show that the failure rate of disc surgery is extremely high—a 50 percent failure rate!

The rate of back surgery in the United States is at least 40 percent higher than in any country in the world, and it is more than five times greater than in England and Scotland. This raises a red flag as to the number of unnecessary disc surgeries being performed in the United States.

Spinal fusion operations are 20 times more common in some states than in others. The rate of disc surgeries in some states per capita can be 50 times higher than in England. This gross discrepancy in disc surgery clearly sends an ominous message that too much disc surgery is being done, and that chiropractors should act as gatekeepers in hospitals, as many back problems can be treated effectively, and many unnecessary back surgeries can be avoided through appropriate chiropractic care.

In January 1976, medical doctors in Los Angeles County went on strike. State audits later concluded that during that month, the death rate **dropped** by more that

153 people, as a result of elective surgeries that were not performed during that month.

Milliman & Robertson, one of the largest actuary and business-consulting firms in America, concluded that *60 percent of all general surgeries are medically unnecessary!*

These kinds of statistics send out a strong message that there is a need for major healthcare reform, with closer inter-professional cooperation between medical doctors and chiropractors.

The Psychological Approach.

The psychological approach involves the use of psychologists, ministers, priests, and rabbis. This is a major category that can apply to many psychological and emotional ailments. The devil manages to squirm himself into many situations, so Christian counseling is often the most appropriate way to correct these problems.

Psychologists tend to attach a bunch of secular names to different abnormal behaviors when the real culprit is frequently the devil. This will be covered in more detail as your read further.

The Chemical or Medical Approach.

If someone has diabetes and needs insulin, or has an open cut and needs to apply an antiseptic to prevent an infection, then the chemical approach is usually appropriate. The human body has its own built-in "drug store" and produces drugs—like antibodies, insulin, hormones, antihistamine, adrenaline, and others—and uses them appropriately.

Government studies show that there is altogether too much over-prescribing of medications, and that many medical patients of today will become the drug addicts of tomorrow. A drug may be compared to a two-edged sword, which can save or take a life. Drug companies spend 18 billion dollars a year promoting drugs, which is far more than they spend on research.

A number of years ago, the U.S. Office of Public Health found that two-thirds of over-the-counter (OTC) drugs do NOT do what their promoters claim. And things are no better today.

Jim Drinkard from *USA Today* wrote that the drug industry owns Congress, the Food and Drug Administration (FDA), the Federal Trade Commission (FTC), and the American Medical Association (AMA). Drinkard noted, "Drugs are sometimes appropriate and, at times, can save a person's life, but they would be well advised to recognize that you should seek natural therapies that address the cause of the disease before choosing a drug-based solution."

In Washington, the drug industry has 1,274 lobbyists—that is more than two lobbyists for every one congressman!

Chuck Grassley, former Chairman of the Senate Finance Committee, observed that, "You can hardly swing a cat by the tail in that town without hitting a pharmaceutical lobbyist."

The Structural/Biomechanical/Manipulative/ Adjustment Approach.

To fully understand what chiropractic is all about and why it is so effective, we need to have a basic understanding of what an incredible body we have and its amazing ability to heal itself, often without drugs and surgery.

Let's begin by examining the anatomy of the spine and its role in healthcare.

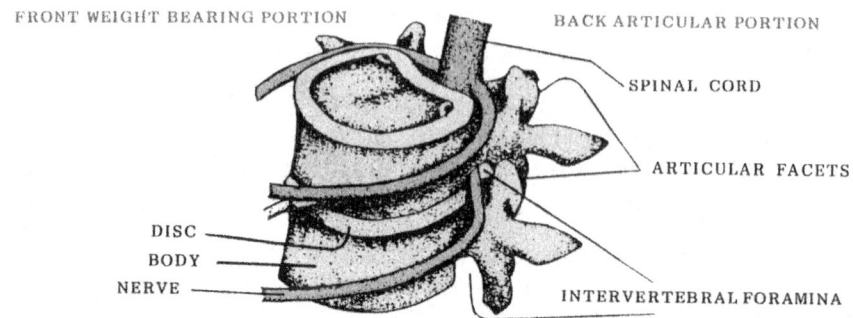

FRONT WEIGHT BEARING PORTION — BACK ARTICULAR PORTION — SPINAL CORD — ARTICULAR FACETS — DISC — BODY — NERVE — INTERVERTEBRAL FORAMINA

The front portion of the spine is weight bearing and consists of vertebral bodies and their discs. The discs are made up of a jelly-like substance enclosed between the vertebrae by fibrous rings. The jelly-like discs act as shock absorbers. If the outer fibrous ring tears and allows some of the jelly to exit its confinement between the vertebrae, you have what they call a "slipped disc."

Some of these conditions may be corrected without surgery by applying traction to the vertebrae, which may suck the jelly back into place, somewhat like a Chinese handcuff. This must be done by a skilled physician, such as a chiropractor or orthopedist. The back portion of the spine gives rise to the joint surfaces, which are called articular facets. They guide and help keep the vertebrae sliding within their normal range of motion.

Small openings are created when the vertebrae sit on top of each other, which allow the nerves and blood vessels to exit.

Impaired function of these nerves can result in a variety of human discomforts, including pain, restricted motion, tenderness, increase in temperature, muscle spasm, shooting pain down the legs or arms, etc. This combination of subjective symptoms (what the patient feels) and objective findings (what the doctor sees) are referred to as a "subluxation complex," or simply called "subluxations" for short.

It is important to note that a "chiropractic subluxation complex" is NOT the same as a medical subluxation, which refers to a dislocation.

If the subluxation is in the upper part of the neck, then neck pain and headaches may result. When it comes to structural and tension headaches, adjustments are in a class by themselves.

If the problem is in the lower neck, then the pain may extend into the arms and all the way down to the fingers. If a subluxation occurs between the shoulder blades, pain may radiate between the ribs to the front of the chest, and may even be mistaken for angina pain.

If the pain is toward the bottom of the spine, then it may cause pain to radiate down the legs and to the toes.

Using drugs to kill the pain, while ignoring the structural cause of the pain, makes no sense at all. It could be compared to smashing a fire alarm and ignoring the fire.

Pain is actually a warning signal telling you that you have a problem that needs to be **corrected** and **NOT masked** with a painkiller.

Spinal adjustments remove these vertebral subluxations, swelling, congestion, and pressure on the nerves, and help to restore normal function. All of this improves nerve activity and allows the body to utilize its natural healing power to function more efficiently.

Chiropractic's great success in the neuro-musculoskeletal field and stress-related ailments and headaches is two-fold. First, it is the result of better training, understanding, and qualification. Second, it represents a rational, safe, and effective approach to structural and biomechanical ailments without the reactions or hazards of drugs or surgery.

The Importance of Structure to Function.

The importance of body structure to function is self-evident everywhere. If we adversely alter the structure of a building, bridge, boat, plane, automobile, locomotive, etc., it will adversely affect their stability and function.

Within the animal kingdom, structure also plays a vital role. Dogs, cats, and other animals, stretch their spines and instinctively seem to know that straightening their spine is beneficial to their well-being.

The same God-given wisdom that created, and maintains this incredible body, also heals it. When we have such an amazing body, we need to respect it and work with it and not work against it.

We need to rely on the safest and most conservative treatments that work *in harmony with our body.*

Chiropractors are not against drugs, but the abusive over-utilization of these drugs promoted by the pharmaceutical industry, which is primarily focused on making money.

The devil also gets into health care by getting control of those pill-oriented patients who become victims of addiction to these pills.

Hippocrates emphasized the importance of the healing power of our God-created nature and instructed, *"Above all, do no harm."* While some doctors may have lost sight of this great wisdom, doctors of chiropractic firmly adhere to this philosophy.

Chapter 2

The Devil Gets into Politics

Prior to the conclusion of the 2012 presidential election, I had written the following material for the second chapter of this book explaining how the devil gets into healthcare, medicine, churches, courts, politics, and families. Governor Mitt Romney had all of the credentials and attributes needed to become one of our greatest presidents, so I was absolutely positive that Governor Romney would easily win the election.

Much to my surprise and shock, Governor Romney lost the election! Rather than rewriting this chapter, I decided to print my original message exactly as I had written it, along with this introductory paragraph explaining that I had written it <u>before</u> the election and let the American people read what might have been. We will see what the next four years will bring. And so, beginning with the next paragraph, here is what I wrote.

* * *

When we see the political state of affairs throughout the world, we know that the devil and his minions are always busy creating all kinds of mischief and divisiveness. But let's just focus on the politics within our nation. We are far better off than in most other countries, and we have every reason to be very proud of America.

When I learned that Mitt Romney would run for president, I began to research the history and

character of the man. One good source to learn about prominent people is from the free Wikipedia; it is a computer encyclopedia. The information given is generally objective and true, and I became very impressed with what I read. I learned that Mitt Romney spent 30 months in France as an unpaid missionary for God, which tells me a lot about the character of the man.

He is a Mormon with a strong Christian faith, and with very high morals and principles. He was born within a wealthy family, but when his father died, he refused to accept one penny of his inheritance and instead donated it to charity. I don't know how many people would do this, because I certainly wouldn't. I doubt that we can find one person in a 1000 who would.

He chose to live in a basement apartment on a tight budget and with little money until he could prove to himself that he had what it took to earn the kind of wealth he acquired, and to do so with honesty and integrity. He became, in the finest sense of the word, a self-made multi-millionaire with very strong Christian principles, and someone you can really trust.

He purchased numerous struggling companies, rebuilt them into successful enterprises, and then sold them at a profit. Christ is not against making money properly, but He also advocates that a percent of our earnings go to God. Romney became very wealthy in the process, and he always donated a large portion of his profits to charity.

If everyone was as giving and generous as Mitt Romney, imagine what a great world it would be to live in, instead of what we have today.

Mitt Romney, realizing that the State of Massachusetts was in economic distress with a three billion dollar deficit, ran for Governor in the state and won the election. After four years, he transformed the state's three billion dollar deficit into a two billion dollar surplus! And he was able to accomplish it with 87 percent of the legislators being Democrats. He was able to cross over the fence politically and unite the two parties. Furthermore, he accepted no salary as governor, which is unprecedented.

We would have to look far and wide to find another such unselfish and giving person. He is one in a million!

Our nation's economic situation has worsened with each passing year during the Obama administration. Unemployment has gone risen every year and people are hurting. It is reaching a crisis level where the interest payments on our loans will soon exceed our national income from taxes. And we certainly do not want to become beholding to the Chinese on a debt that we cannot pay, while the Obama administration is putting us deeper into debt every day.

Many Americans are grossly unaware of the dire consequences of becoming financially obligated to China, and it is foolish to expect that the Chinese will ever forgive the loan. Only Americans are forgiving on matters like these. We would become obligated to China and the consequences are unthinkable.

I was delighted to hear that our nation was going to get a new president, and that Mitt Romney was the obvious choice. He is both a unifier and skillful repairman with a history of repairing companies and states, and I feel that his presidency is an answer to our prayers, and that the election should be a slam-dunk.

However, I began to hear on the news that Mitt Romney was actually trailing in the polls, and that if the election was held today, he would lose. I was astounded by this! How could this be true? Why should we keep the same president with broken promises and a failing record for nearly four years, especially when we have another candidate with superior qualifications and a great track record of repairing distressed companies and even saving a state. It just didn't make any sense to me.

And then the answer surfaced. The Democratic Party was spending millions of dollars on a smear campaign to make Governor Romney appear like an evil, uncaring, and ruthless scoundrel. They were involved in a major character assassination of Romney, but the Democratic Party had to know that they were lying. Nobody can be so naïve as to the truth.

The Democrats were pulling out all the stops to get Obama reelected with outrageous lies, while the devil was in all his glory instigating a false image of a decent Christian human being who was only trying to save his nation from an impending economic tragedy.

Mitt Romney's campaigning certainly was not about himself, as he had absolutely nothing to gain; he is independently wealthy, while his history shows that he is a kind, giving and generous humanitarian.

I have lived through 15 presidential elections where I have supported both parties, but this presidential election was by far the most dishonest and vicious campaign that I have ever witnessed. I am politically independent and have supported legislators on both sides of the fence.

The laws to protect people from defamation and slander do not apply to political elections. Obviously, if the defamatory and slander laws applied to political campaigning, the election would get so bogged down with lawsuits and counter-lawsuits that it would never take place. This gives the devil and his cooperating accomplices—in this instance, the Democrats—opportunity to use lies and character assassination. The devil is in all of his glory.

We can call it devil guidance and intervention, or supernatural evil influence, but whatever you want to call it—it has happened! The Democratic Party even wanted to remove God from their platform. This was the last straw.

I was furious by what was happening and I prepared 16 reasons why we must elect Mitt Romney. I ran full page ads in seven of our local suburban newspapers, as well as in the largest Polish ethnic daily newspaper in America, which is based in Chicago, and which circulates newspapers to subscribers in over 30 states.

The ad will repeat some information I have already covered here, but it bears repeating, because it sends a strong message as to how the devil can get into the minds of people. The following ad speaks for itself.

"Sixteen Reasons Why Governor Romney Must Become President"

Governor Romney is an unselfish, compassionate, humanitarian and contributor. He is deeply concerned about the self-destructive direction our country is going in and he wants to save our country. He is truly a man of God. He cannot speak openly about his many charitable donations or contributions because when you give, you don't announce it publicly by blowing trumpets like the hypocrites.

Since Governor Romney will not tell people about his many charitable donations and contributions to America, will you inform your family, friends, and neighbors?

1. Governor Romney took over the Olympics program, which was in serious trouble, turned it into an outstanding success, and did not accept one penny for his contribution. Everyone who had contact with Governor Romney said he was a highly qualified manager and a man of integrity.

2. As Governor of Massachusetts, and after four years in office, he removed a three billion dollar debt and turned it into a two billion dollar surplus. And he did not accept <u>one penny of compensation</u> for serving as the Governor of Massachusetts.

3. Governor Romney took troubled companies and turned them into successful enterprises, creating new jobs. He can apply this same expertise to our nation and rebuild it. He started STAPLES, which now has 2,000 stores and provides 90,000 jobs.

4. He was an unpaid volunteer for his father's gubernatorial campaign.

5. He was an unpaid volunteer intern in his father's governor's office for eight years.

6. He was an unpaid bishop and state president of his church for 10 years—a true Christian.

7. He was an unpaid president of the Salt Lake Olympic Committee for three years.

8. Gov. Romney gave his entire inheritance to charity and went to Utah with his own money to prove what he could do. His incredible skill made him one of America's wealthiest self-made millionaires. In 2011, he gave over $4M to Charity—almost 19% of his income. He is a major unselfish contributor to society—someone we can be proud to have as a president. <u>(By comparison, President Obama, who is worth $10M, gave one% to charity, and Biden gave $300 or 0.0013%)</u>.

31

9. Governor Romney served as a missionary in France for 30 months and was a strong advocate for his church to allow blacks to become ministers. When he finally heard it announced on his car radio, he pulled over off the road and wept with joy for them. This needs to be brought out to everyone, especially black Americans.

10. At least we know what religion Governor Romney is, and that he won't desecrate our flag, bow down to foreign powers, or practice fiscal irresponsibility. And, he can turn the financial debacle of the current administration into an economically stable one. If Romney wins the election, history will show him as one of our greatest presidents who saved our country.

11. He never smoked pot, took drugs, never got drunk, did not associate with communists and terrorists, nor did he attend a church whose pastor called for God to damn the United States.

12. We see the election as almost being between good and evil, and how we are being given a new leader who is a strong Christian and missionary with great integrity, who has a solid record of rebuilding broken companies, and is noted for saving Massachusetts from bankruptcy—and he did it without accepting one penny for being governor. He is a highly skilled organizer and builder. This is what America desperately needs!

    Regarding Governor Romney's Mormon faith, the Bible is perfect, but churches are not. There are 41,000 different Presbyterian denominations all for one God, which tells us that while the Bible is perfect, churches, are not.

13. Meanwhile, President Obama presents a history of gross incompetence, cover-ups, lies, and damnable lies, passing the buck, broken promises,

discouraging independence, punishing success, promoting dependency, non-transparency, cronyism, disingenuous conduct and hypocrisy, demagoguery by turning his back on Christians and Jews while pampering, pandering and apologizing to the radical Muslims as they destroyed our embassy and killed our ambassador.

14. The last election proved that most American people are NOT prejudiced by <u>voting in</u> a black man as president, but in this election, they must now prove that they are not foolish and gullible by <u>voting him out</u>!

15. The majority of the Democratic delegates incredibly wanted to remove God from their platform. These Democratic delegates deserve to be called Demon-crats!

16. The house unanimously rejected Obama's irresponsible budget by a vote of 414-0. Running a country without a budget is both unprecedented and inexcusable. We cannot afford four more years of Obama's "borrow and spend" policies. The borrower becomes a slave to the lender.

Our founding fathers wanted to remove politics from religion—not remove religion from politics. Fifty-six of our Founding Fathers had Bible school degrees as ministers, and our Capital building was once a mega church with thousands of people worshiping there every week. Four of the paintings within the Capital deal with Christian history. Thomas Jefferson, who was the least religious within the group, had Congress print and endorse the first English written Bible in America, recommending its use in schools, and for all of its inhabitants.

And America grew by leaps and bounds. The U.S. Marine Corps Band even played worship music in the Capital building.

Today, we see God being driven out of everywhere. Hence, I have written a book entitled, *The Case for Christ and Against the Devil.* It is available from Amazon and Kindle. See www.chetwilk.com video documentary with Hugh Downs for INSIGHT. I was voted one of the three most respected chiropractors in America after winning a landmark antitrust lawsuit against the American Medical Association." (End of ad)

I sent the above information to eight different newspapers as a full-page ad, which included the largest, *Polish Daily News*, which is a subscription publication that is read in over 30 states. My local Park Ridge newspaper chose to put the above ad on page two, right after the cover page.

The following information was submitted to my copyeditor PRIOR TO THE ELECTION and she did the appropriate editing and sent it back to me, which I include here.

I knew that I had to write another book, which classically brings out how the devil gets into politics and literally takes over the minds of people. When the first debate was held between Governor Romney and President Obama, our nation saw the real Governor Romney and not the ugly monster the Democrats had portrayed him as. They recognized a genuine, sincere, caring, supremely qualified, compassionate, knowledgeable, articulate, honest, professorial, and presidential-looking man running for president, and everyone watching realized the truth. All of the ugly propaganda and millions of dollars spent to attack this man were blown away within 90 minutes of the debate. And everyone agreed—Democrats and Republicans alike—the debate was no contest. Since that first debate, the polls have gradually moved toward Mitt Romney and he single-handedly won the debate.

The Obama administration has done little to advance the Afro-American people, except to

encourage dependence on big government. But this only creates the kind of dependency that Dr. Martin Luther King was trying to eliminate; he wanted to make them completely free and not dependent on government handouts and food stamps.

Dependency is not what made America great, and this is why everyone wants to come to America to reside. It is for the opportunity to become free and independent from the government. It should be our churches that should be able to pitch in and help the unfortunate victims, rather than relying on the state for help. This should be the role of the churches and charitable organizations like the Salvation Army, who are available to help the less fortunate people. Ninety-six percent of the money that is given to the Salvation Army goes toward helping the needy, which is unprecedented in America, and which is why it is my favorite charitable organization.

I would be remiss if I did not include The American Legion, Veterans of Foreign Wars, Disabled American Veterans, Military Order of Purple Hearts, Vietnam Veterans Association, Make a Wish, St. Jude Research Hospital, Wounded Warriors Project, and Ronald McDonald Houses.

A calculation of 26 major civil rights votes from 1933 through the 1960's Civil Rights Era shows that Republicans favored civil rights in approximately 96 percent of the votes, whereas the Democrats *opposed* them in 80 percent of the votes! These facts have been intentionally overlooked by the leftwing Democrats for an obvious reason. It is interesting to note that Afro-Americans overwhelmingly vote for Democrats.

The devil knows when and how to take sides and manipulate people (and parties) to create turmoil and divisiveness. See *"The Democratic Party's Long and Shameful History of Bigotry and Racism"* on your computer. Every Afro-American person should read it on the Internet and become better enlightened. And by the way, it was Abraham Lincoln who fought to free the slaves and paid the ultimate price for it—and he was a Republican.

The liberal media kept bringing up how much money Mitt Romney has just to invoke class envy. There was no other reason for doing it. Envy is one of the devil's tools, and he uses it effectively. Meanwhile, the same liberal media avoids mentioning the wealth of Democratic presidential candidates like John Kerry or John Edwards, how they obtained their wealth, and it certainly was not like the honorable and constructive way that Governor Romney did it.

The Bible tells us that before the end time comes, we will witness all kinds of disasters. It is interesting to note that the worst natural disaster in modern history came on the heels of the most vicious and dishonest political campaign in American history, hitting one of the strongholds of the Democratic Party.

It gives us good reason to become better Christians and to listen to the teachings of the Apostle Paul who faced all kinds of horrific adversities, yet never once questioned God. Adversity is given to us so that it can make us stronger and better, just like it did for the Apostle Paul.

Repairing our battered Northeast will take a lot of hard work, patience, and determination, but you can be sure that our new president will surround himself with some of the finest talent who will be working in a bi-partisan way, and we will prevail in this crisis. And, if anyone blames God for what has been happening, they will play right into the hands of the devil.

An important requirement of any good politician is that he must be flexible and willing to step across the aisle and change his position in the best interest of the nation.

The only person who has never changed His mind or made a mistake was crucified 2,000 years ago. It takes a fair-minded politician to acknowledge that he is not perfect and that he may have to alter his position if circumstances demand it. To criticize or attack this flexibility and call it "flip-flopping" is counterproductive to our nation and comes from the evil one, who is a divider.

Politicians who never change their minds in spite of overwhelming evidence to change course, become unreasonable, hardheaded obstructionists, and only divide a nation. This is exactly what we have witnessed between 2008 and 2012 in Washington. President Obama's budget was rejected in the House by a 114-0 vote and the Senate rejected it by 0-90. President Obama did not get one Democratic vote. This says it all. It should be a learning lesson for everybody.

One of my favorite politicians is Harry Truman, and I'll bet if he met Mitt Romney that the two of them would hit it off beautifully. And, I would add John F. Kennedy and Ronald Reagan to this group. What a dynamic foursome they would make!

I believe the day will come when history will show that Mitt Romney will be ranked very high amongst our greatest presidents. He will have saved America from a major fiscal disaster.

I cite what has happened in this election, because it provides a classic example of how the devil can get into any place that he chooses to create divisiveness and hatred. My attack is on the devil and not any political party. The devil will always choose whomever best serves his wicked ways and, in this instance, he happened to choose the Democrats.

The above information was written PRIOR to the presidential election and the following was written AFTER the presidential election.

* * *

There is an old saying that all is fair at love and war, and I would add politics to this list. There is a prevailing attitude in American politics that it's all about winning and not about how the win was achieved, whether it was won honestly or fraudulently.

As early as February of 2012, the democrats spent 17 million dollars on a vicious character assignation of Governor Romney, yet in our society's mindset, the president won fair and square.

In my mind, and I'm sure in God's eyes, it was an ill-gotten victory of which they cannot be proud.

Hence, the term "dirty politics" has become an accepted way of life and no one generally seems to care.

Winston Churchill said the difference between war and politics is that in war you are killed and die but once, but in politics, you are killed many times.

The Democratic Party even wanted to remove God from its platform, which I thought would arouse a reaction from our Christian community, but no one seemed to care. Where were the Christians? Had they responded appropriately, the outcome of the election would have been reversed.

And there was a question of transparency and whether or not President Obama was actually an American citizen, but again the general public really didn't care.

Donald Trump, who is a great American and a living icon, generously offered to donate five million dollars to go to the charity of the president's choice, if he would simply release his school records and birth certificate. Was he a foreign exchange student? Obama did not release them.

Is anyone even curious as to why he withheld his records? This money could have helped poor people living in poverty. Is there anything wrong with what Donald Trump did? The president even made a joke out of it on a late night talk show, while the audience laughed. It doesn't speak well for America. It shows the kind of public apathy and indifference that can undermine a nation. More importantly, it is an attitude that can destroy a nation.

We have seen many natural disasters and flooding, which have been prophesied in the Bible. God was sending us all kinds of warnings, and again the general public attitude was oblivious to these happenings.

We were experiencing the devil's weapons of public indifference, ignorance, complacency, and apathy on matters we should be acutely concerned about. But, once again, no one generally seemed to care. Satan was using these weapons and he was very much in charge.

Our nation is falling into a pattern attributed to the Scottish professor, lawyer, and writer Alexander Tytler spoke about way back when we had 13 states:

> **"A democracy cannot exist as a permanent form of government. It can only exist until the voters discover that they can vote themselves money from the public treasure. From that moment on, the majority always votes for the candidates promising the most money from the public treasury, with the result that a democracy collapses over loose fiscal policy, followed by a dictatorship. The average age of the world's great civilizations has been 200 years. These nations have progressed through the following sequence:**

from bondage to spiritual faith, from spiritual faith to great courage, from courage to liberty, from liberty to abundance, from abundance to selfishness, from selfishness to complacency, from complacency to apathy, from apathy to dependence, from dependency back to bondage."

As our president will try to establish some kind of legacy for himself, I need not tell you where we are heading if he does not change his course. Four more years of doing the same thing will be fatal to America.

Einstein said that doing the same thing over and over again and expecting a different result is insanity. In the past four years, President Obama spent more money than *every other president combined* since President Washington, and he wants a "blank check" to spend *more* money, which will unquestionably destroy America economically. It will make us beholding to China.

Spending beyond our means is generally viewed as irresponsibility and stupidity, but I do NOT see it as such. I see it as how the devil was able get into the minds of million of citizens to deliberately divide and hurt America economically. President Obama was a senator, and senators simply do not have the negotiating experience of a governor. I recall speaking with Senator McGovern, who unsuccessfully ran for president, and he told me that after leaving politics, he went into business—and he bankrupted! He was going to try to run our government and couldn't even run his own business. And then he told me that the reason he bankrupted was because of "too many government regulations."

Governor Romney started out as a governor and was an extremely successful one. He felt that with his past record of bailing out Massachusetts and converting many companies into major successes, that he could save America. He is a private person who did not seek public attention and who had no desire to run for president, according to his family. He would have happily stepped aside if he saw someone else who could have done the job. He is the true hero and tragedy of what might have been.

The greatness of a man needs to be measured beyond his presidency. After Truman retired, he was offered a corporate position with a great salary. He declined the offer saying, "You don't want me. You want the office of the president, and that doesn't belong to me. It belongs to the American people and it's not for sale."

Truman said he spent the first six months in office wondering how he ever got where he was. Then he said he spent the rest of his time wondering how all the other politicians ever got where they were.

Congress wanted to give President Truman the Congressional Metal of Honor on his 87th birthday, but he declined saying, "I don't consider that I have done anything that should be the reason for any award, Congressional or otherwise."

President Truman paid for his own stamps and licked them, and paid for his own travel expenses and food. He retired in the same home he had lived in throughout his life, and with a U.S. Army pension of $13,507.72.

Modern politicians have found a new level of success by cashing in on the presidency, creating untold wealth. Political offices are even up for sale, as we have seen in Illinois.

Good old Harry Truman was right when he observed, "My choices in life were either to play the piano in a whore house or be a politician, and to tell the truth, there's hardly any difference."

And as far as passing the buck goes, as too many politicians have done, he said the buck stopped with him. Now that's a true public servant! I suggest that we dig him up and clone him!

Our future politicians, regardless of their political party, need to be a lot more "in their face" if any opponent tries to lie, cover-up or obfuscate the issues. Harry Truman brought a classic example of this when he said, "I don't give them hell. I just tell the truth and they think it's hell!" He was my kind of guy and a straight shooter. And, by the way, he won! I hope that we all have learned a lesson from him.

President Obama said that we have the greatest nation in the world, and then almost in the same breath added that he was going to change it. But most of us will not like the kind of change to which he refers. We are spending 1.3 trillion dollars more per year than our government takes in, and there is no sign that this will change. We need to trim the unnecessary and wasteful pork barrel spending. Raising taxes while not eliminating the worthless and foolish pork barrel spending will be like giving drugs to a drug addict or alcohol to an alcoholic. We'll get deeper and deeper into dependency to our creditors, like China.

The Bible says that the borrower becomes a slave to the lender. Lest we wake up to this reality, the consequences will be devastating. I believe that the devil is leading our nation using selfishness, indifference, apathy, and too much dependency on big government. And, if we don't change our course, it will be the end of America as we know it, and to our two-party system.

* * *

The devil is a very deceptive and conniving person, which gives him incredible influence. The devil has been able to convince an entire nation to sit back and do nothing, while every 14 minutes someone dies from taking unnecessary prescription medications. This is a modern day medical holocaust!

Meanwhile, the medical profession acknowledges in their journals that they indeed are killing 3,000 every week! It is by their own admission. If this were a terrorist group killing 3,000 people every week everybody would be up in arms. Why isn't America up in arms now? Again, the devil did it. His weapon is greed.

We can look down our noses and say how foolish or misguided the extremist radical Muslims are to believe that by strapping bombs to their children or flying planes into a buildings, that it will get them into heaven. The devil has obliviously been able to get into these Muslims.

But who is more foolish or misguided, the American people who are killing themselves at the rate of 3,000 every week with **unnecessary** drugs and surgery, or the radical Muslims who kill themselves in a different manner? What is the difference? They are both irrational and stupid acts, yet they take place on a regular basis because people are being deceived by the devil.

This is not a matter of foolishness or bad judgment, but a matter of how convincing the devil can be and get away with murder, and do it without being exposed! Sixty percent of the Christians do not believe that the devil exists in spite of how Christ clearly said that there IS a devil! Our churches need to do a better job of educating their congregations about the devil.

The devil was able to convince a majority of the democratic delegates to remove God from their platform, but our churches were not allowed to caution their members about this anti-Christian act. This is terribly wrong. We need more religion in politics.

The radical Muslims are called Shiites, and they represent 10 to 15 percent of their population. The 85 to 90 percent are Sunnis, who are peace loving and non-aggressive people that do not represent any threat to our society. However, there are 200 million Shiite Muslims willing to kill themselves and others, while our president and many of our political leaders are not taking them seriously. The Shiites actually hate the Sunnis, which is like our far left liberal counterparts who dislike conservatives.

Our president insists that the Muslims do not represent any serious threat to America, but he is mistaken.

Most of the Shiites, or about 80 percent of them live in Iran, and their leaders openly indicate that their intent is to destroy Israel. They present a major problem to the world.

God has given me an assignment to provide solid evidence to the world that there is a God in heaven and a devil in hell, and to create more awareness as to how the devil works. Proving the devil is real is a very challenging responsibility, but I have absolute and conclusive evidence beyond all reasonable doubt, which you will see as you read on.

Chapter 3

How the Devil Gets into Churches

Satan loves to get into churches; it is one of his favorite haunts. He wants to be like the Most High. If he can get into a pastor, he puts the entire congregation at risk, and the minister will commit some un-Christian-like conduct, while Satan will be working diligently to convince him, and everyone else around him, that what they are doing is proper.

Many Christians believe that the devil is not real, but only a symbol of evil. Either the churches are not doing their job of making their members realize that the devil does exist and is a real person, or the devil is getting into the churches and preventing pastors from preaching the truth about the devil's existence.

One of the devil's weapons is gossip. If you have heard it in your church, it is a clear indication that the devil was behind it. It's a dead giveaway.

The devil's modus operendi is to work covertly and not be exposed, and he has to have an astronomical I.Q. and thousands years of experience. He is real and I can back it up with very strong evidence.

One of the advantages of beating an enemy in combat is knowing their personality. I read a military combat manual from WWII, which described the personalities of different nations. The Germans would follow the orders of their officers down to the last survivor.

The Italians and French were less committed to follow orders from their superiors. The Norwegians were slow to ire, but once they were, you had better get out of their way. Meanwhile, the American soldiers were the most dangerous, because no one ever knew what crazy or imaginative thing they might do, or come up while in combat.

Since America is a melting pot made up of all kinds of ethnic peoples, American soldiers are unpredictable in combat. And if someone doesn't believe that the devil is genuine, they become an easier target for him to conquer.

One of Satan's strategies is to insult and label Christians who believe the devil is real, as being religious fanatics or members of the lunatic fringe. The Bible makes it crystal clear that there is a devil in hell.

Satan is mentioned about 19 times in the *Old Testament* and 15 times in the *New Testament*. He is real, and if we don't believe Christ and the Bible, then whom can we believe?

Let me begin with a classic example of how the devil worked through the churches and sabotaged my long-time marriage.

Wanting to mend things with my wife, Ardith, I asked my minister in Park Ridge, IL, to urge her to return home for marriage counseling. She was residing in Encinitas, California at the time.

I was shocked and disappointed to learn that my minister had actually complimented Ardith for leaving me, and then refused to urge her to return home for Christian counseling. I was stunned with disbelief that a man professing to be an ordained minister could possibly do something like this. He took sides and made the judgment that my wife was right in leaving me without speaking to both of us and hearing the facts. I have the letters to back up that what I am saying is true.

I had sent my minister extensive information about our marital situation, so he was not entirely ignorant about our case, but there was absolutely no reason for him to take such a wrongful position and refuse to suggest couple's marital counseling. We had been happily married for over 40 years. It was totally inexcusable. It was not the Christian thing to do.

The only reason the minister gave for his inappropriate position was that it was "personal and confidential," which was not an answer.

Dr. Warren W. Wiersbe, a "**pastor's pastor,**" and author of more than 100 books wrote, ***The Strategy of Satan: How to Detect and Defeat Him.*** He said, "Simply because a preacher is a professed Christian, a moral man, and a graduate of a seminary, does not mean he is truly saved and a servant of Jesus Christ.

I believe Dr. Wiersbe's words apply to my ex-wife, Ardith's behavior. She read the Bible every day and went to church every Sunday, but even being a devout Christian does not mean that one cannot become the devil's victim, which I believe Ardith is. Satan has thousands of years of experience in deception and anyone can be a victim <u>if they underestimate the devil</u>. Ardith's sudden switch from being a loving wife to suddenly leaving me, and then refusing to consider couple's counseling, proves this point.

What else besides the devil could cause such an abrupt change of heart after so many years together?

Dr. Wiersbe noted how many churches put new Christians into places of leadership without allowing them to mature in areas of lesser ministry, and so they may become conceited and not have a forgiving spirit, which opens the door for Satan to enter. I believe this is what happened with my Park Ridge church and its youthful minister. His inappropriate letter to me and disgraceful advice to Ardith proves my point.

Pastor Wiersbe's solution for when the devil gets into a church is, "Let every church member—and spiritual leaders in particular—learn to detect and defeat Satan. We must practice speaking the truth in love. **(Ephesians 4:15)** We must forgive one another and learn to use the wisdom that is from above. Whenever there is a division, we must wait on the Lord for spiritual unity. If unity does not come, we must discover who the people are that Satan is using to hinder the work, and we must deal with them in firmness and love. I know personally how difficult this is, but I also know the blessings and joys that can come when Satan has been evicted."

I was trying to save a marriage, which every Christian minister should support. I explained to him that Ardith did not have to live with me during the marriage counseling, and did not even have to see me while she was there, and that she could stay at an undisclosed location.

I loved my wife. All I wanted was the opportunity for each of us to talk things out with a spiritual advisor, so that we would have a chance at reconciliation.

Still, the minister refused to reverse his position, and even sent me a letter telling me not to contact him any further and to not attend his church.

This supposed Christian leader actually judged me without even knowing me, advised my wife to forego counseling, and then even banned me from attending his church. I was astounded.

The letter, which I have on file, was signed by this young, junior minister, and co-signed by the church's senior minister and Chairman of the Board, which was somewhat defamatory. The chairman of the church board had never met me nor had he even spoke to me, yet he cosigned the letter.

I then asked to have a meeting with the church board members, but, again, was refused. It is totally inappropriate for any church to refuse a conference with a member. It was like a conspiracy and cover-up for the junior minister. This had to be the devil's influence.

I called the church and asked the secretary for their e-mail address so I could send them a letter appealing for their help. The secretary recognized my name, refused to give it to me, and said if I emailed it, she wouldn't open it anyway. The entire church staff was infected by the devil.

Ardith had no moral basis for leaving me. I was faithful to her. There was no mental or physical cruelty, no womanizing, drugs, alcohol, or lack of support, and she cannot say I was not generous to a fault with her and my daughters. I was at a total loss as to why my wife decided to leave me. I wanted answers and a chance to mend things between us. I wanted a chance for our mutual faith to bring us back together.

It is a disgrace for any church to compliment a woman for leaving her husband without a cause, and then refuse to suggest marriage counseling. It is wrong by every standard. The issue is larger than me; it's a matter of churches behaving in inappropriate, non-Christian ways. I had heard stories about how the devil gets into churches, and here I was experiencing it within my very own church.

Ardith had vacillated about returning home, and at one point, she even called me on the telephone and left a message on my answering machine, asking me to "Sweep her off her feet and bring her home," but then changed her mind the very next day. I was confused. She was confused. We needed help, but we didn't get it.

I believe that Ardith and I were victims in a spiritual war, and the guidance Ardith was receiving from her church was anything but Christian. This had to be the devil's influence.

Ardith and I needed appropriate Christian counseling, but we did not receive it from her former church minister in Park Ridge or from her church minister in Encinitas, California.

The devil was covering all of his bases.

Ardith's so-called Christian marriage counselor had been recommended by her church in Encinitas, California, but he refused to recommend that she return to Chicago for marriage counseling. The excuse he gave was that he was only focusing on her nervous condition and not on her marriage problems, which was bogus and inexcusable. It would be like a physician saying he was only focusing on Ardith's stomach problem, while ignoring the cancer on her foot.

When I told this to her counselor over the phone, he told Ardith that he could no longer counsel her because he'd be looking over his shoulder. I'd be looking over my shoulder too, if I had given such bad advice. He also realized that I would no longer be sending him checks for her counseling.

The only logical answer was that he did not want to lose her as a paying client, and making money seemed more important to him than giving appropriate advice to his client.

The devil's weapon is greed, which is at the root of many evils.

It is well established that appropriate marriage counseling requires that both parties be counseled by the same counselor or counselors, which could only be done properly in Chicago, and not with Ardith living over 2,000 miles away. The Encinitas marriage counselor was dead wrong and he knew it.

The two most critical Christian individuals, an ordained minister and so-called Christian counselor, who could have influenced Ardith, refused to help her, and they let her down. They also let me down.

I reported the marriage counselor to the Board of Psychology, which actually recommended that Ardith file the complaint against her counselor because I could not do it as a third party. The board knew I had a good case against the counselor, but without Ardith's authorization, the board was prevented from taking action against him.

I sent several letters explaining all of the facts about our marriage, as well as my book, to the senior pastor at Ardith's church in Encinitas, California, hoping that as a Christian, he would have integrity and understand my intentions, but I never got an answer to my mail.

There was a group of local Park Ridge ministers who got together on a monthly basis, and so I requested that I be permitted to attend their meeting to discuss my situation. After sending letters to all of the local ministers in Park Ridge, not one responded to my mail. Maybe my letters were too emotional or maybe too adamant, but I was heartbroken and seeking help. It was devastating to be turned down by my own church leaders when I was simply asking to be heard, to discuss what was happening in my life, and to gain some understanding. At the time, I didn't realize how thorough the devil could be.

Then great Civil Rights leader Dr Martin Luther King said, "He who accepts evil without protesting against it is really cooperating with it." I share his passion by fighting evil in any form, whether it is in medicine or politics, but especially when it is in churches. There is nothing worse than a hypocritical minister.

Churches are supposed to support marriages and not stonewall someone who is trying to save a marriage, and especially when that person had a legitimate reason for speaking out. And when all of the churches that were contacted turned a blind eye and deaf ear to what was being said, it brings to mind those words of Martin Luther King.

Two years later, I returned to my former church and the minister was now the senior minister. He refused to even face me and instead had one of his assistants tell me, "It is all over, move on, find another wife." This kind of talk has no place within a church. It goes right into the face of Christ and the Bible.

Christ said that no man should split what God has joined together.

The real issue here is not that it happened to me, but that it should not happen to anyone. It does not speak well for all of these churches that have chosen to remain silent.

If a physician is guilty of medical malpractice of equal seriousness as to what my Park Ridge minister committed on a spiritual level, the physician would be called before a disciplinary committee and face disciplinary measures, if not even have his license suspended or revoked.

A minister on the other hand, can get away with this kind of ill conduct and stonewall people as other ministers simply look the other way, and choose not to become involved. This is hardly a Christian attitude and, I believe the devil played a role in these cases.

The Bible is perfect, but churches and ministers are not. I do not attend church on a regular basis, but only on occasion, and I think this is true of most Christians. But I have God with me 7 days a week and 24 hours a day, and this is where it counts.

The founding fathers of our nation wanted to take politics out of churches, not religion out of politics, while the devil cleverly perverted the intent of our founding fathers.

We need more religion in politics and the decency and fair play that Christ can bring into public service. We may see less of the kind of mean-spirited lies and vicious character assassinations we witnessed of a fine and decent Christian man like Mitt Romney, who I firmly believe could have unified and healed our divided nation.

He's had setbacks in life, but so did Abraham Lincoln. Still, in my mind, he is a genuine American hero, and my heart goes out to him and what might have been.

The presidential race was virtually a tie, and had the democrats, (or shall I say demon-crats), not spent 17 million dollars early in the race defaming Governor Romney with blatant lies, he most assuredly would have won the election. It is therefore obvious that this was an ill-gotten victory and a tragic loss for our great country.

Senator McCain said that President Obama's presidency was won 'fair and square." In my mind, it was unfair and crooked. If the character assassinations were spoken or written anywhere else, other than in an election, Governor Romney would have justification for some serious slander and defamation charges. It is sad to see how we have allowed our politics to crawl so low into the gutter that we can refer to it as "fair and square."

I wonder how the Good Lord will look upon what has happened. We need to desperately pray for America. It needs all the help it can get.

I am absolutely convinced that before you finish reading this book, you will realize the existence of the devil as being real. It is an easy read and not too lengthy, so you can finish it in little time, and I <u>guarantee you</u> that it will change your thinking on the subject.

Read this book to the finish with an open mind (as opposed to an empty head), because what you will read will greatly surprise and impress you, and be important to you and your family in many ways. And you'll be glad you did.

Chapter 4

How the Devil Destroys Families

Anybody would be especially proud to have a family like mine. My wife, Ardith, was a scrub nurse with a top-notch team of surgeons led by Dr. Willis Potts of Children's Memorial Hospital. She was a devoted Christian who spent the first hour of every morning reading her Bible.

After we started a family, Ardith became totally devoted to our children. I did not want her to get a job so that she could be a full-time mom.

I have three daughters. My oldest girl, Kim, was very popular in high school. She was co-captain of the cheerleaders and was chosen Spirit Queen at Maine South High School. I would watch Kim cheerleading during games and I couldn't help but be very proud of her. She stood out in the crowd. The school principal even noted to me what a great role model she was, and how she carried her responsibility with a lot of class.

After high school, Kim became a champion tri-athlete and accumulated a closet full of first-place State Championship trophies, including the huge annual triathlon held downtown in Chicago in 1989, where she won "**First Place Individual Female.**"

I proudly display her trophy in my office reception room. She left all her trophies behind and didn't care for them.

Kim has the courage and tenacity of a bull, and when she sets a goal, she pursues it relentlessly. She was invited to the world-famous *Iron Man Triathlon* in Hawaii, which consists of 2.4-mile swim, 112-mile bike, and 26-mile marathon, and she finished among the top contenders.

She was also in the *Auburn Triathlon* in California, which is considered to be even tougher than the *Iron Man Triathlon.* It required riding up and down steep hills on a bike, at times going 50 miles an hour, with dangerous crosswinds.

The running portion of the race required running and crawling up and down steep hills, sometimes on all fours. At one point, they pedaled uphill for 11 miles non-stop. It was more like an obstacle course. Only 24 hardy and courageous women entered this race, and Kim finished among the top leaders.

Kim became a firefighter in Denver. Trainees have to carry a 150-pound dummy up a ladder and Kim scored higher than some of the men in her class, which was incredible, because she is a petite woman. While working as a firefighter, she wanted to become a part-time teacher for handicapped children on her days off from the Fire Department.

You can imagine the kind of inspiration Kim can be to handicapped children, being tutored by a champion tri-athlete and firefighter. Firefighters enjoy greater public respect than physicians. I encouraged Kim to go on with becoming a teacher.

Can there be a greater Christian contribution to helping others than tutoring and inspiring handicapped children as a champion tri-athlete and firefighter?

To say Kim was an outstanding contributor would be an understatement. I often speak about how proud I am of her commitment and persistence in life to be the best that she can be.

My youngest daughter, Cindy, put herself through her last two years of college by working two jobs, and she carried a straight "A" average.

She became a special education teacher for troubled children and chose to teach in a tough inner-city neighborhood in Chicago her first year, while her mother and I worried about her safety. Cindy had a difficult time in high school with her studies, so she could relate to these children. She would purchase treats for her students as an incentive, even though she had little herself.

While teaching special education in the inner city of Chicago, she decided to study the Italian language. A year later, she went to Italy by herself, which took a lot of courage, going to a new country and not even knowing if she could find work to survive. She was alone and almost penniless, but found employment, which provided her with lodgings and she traveled throughout Europe.

After she was there for one year, she was offered a position teaching English, but decided it was time to return to America and she chose California as her new home.

I had an opportunity to observe Cindy while she was teaching in California and she was outstanding. As the students entered her classroom, and later as they left, they would hug Cindy affectionately.

You could see the love, affection, and wonderful chemistry she had with all of her students. Special education teachers often get "burned out" because it is a highly demanding job, and so Cindy decided to take time off from teaching for a while.

She opened a coffee shop and committed herself to an enormous $7,500-a-month lease, and worked 12 hours a day to make it into a success. She hoped to get her sisters to become partners with her in the coffee shop, but they declined.

It took a lot of courage and commitment to take on such a huge financial obligation, because if she had not succeeded in paying this huge rent, she could have lost her home and everything she had.

Later, Cindy sold her coffee shop and returned to teaching. With her ability, understanding, and compassion for these children, she could open her own school and become very much in demand.

Cindy is also a great entrepreneur. She found a condominium she liked in La Jolla, and so I gave her money for a down payment. She lived in the condo while she fixed it up, and used her first condo as collateral to purchase a second condo. Within a very short time, she parlayed both of her condos into a beautiful home in Encinitas, California. I often spoke to my patients and friends about her entrepreneurial genius, and how proud I was of her.

Cathy is my middle daughter. She chose to become a beautician to help support her family, and she put herself through Beauty College while raising her daughter. She is the only daughter who made me a proud grandpa.

All three of my daughters are model citizens who never took drugs, didn't smoke, and never got into any trouble with the law.

How could I not be extremely proud of all three of them?

At home in my private office, I keep photographs of my wife and three daughters, and plaques that they each made for me, which I cherish.

Cathy made a plaque for me that said, in part:

"He is my hero . . .

He is always at my side . . .

He is always there for me . . .

He is there to pick me up when I am down . . .

My hero is thoughtful and kind . . .

My hero is great; it's me who's proud . . .

My hero is my dad, I'm glad to say."

Cathy's loving plaque is on the wall of my private office, right above my computer, so I can see it every day as I sit at the computer.

Next to Cathy's plaque is one made by Cindy, with a large red heart and a message over the heart, which says: *"I love my father."* And I certainly love Cindy.

Cindy also gave me a booklet entitled *A Special Kind of Love.* It was about a man who had a special way to tell his son, *"I love you."* Cindy crossed out the *"son"* throughout the booklet and replaced it with *"daughter."*

She autographed the booklet with: **"To Dad, Happy Father's Day! Thanks for being supportive over the past few years. You're the greatest – I mean it. Love, Cindy, your daughter."** This was on Father's day in June of 1997.

On the opposite wall of my private office is a composite of many childhood photos of Kim and me, and on the bottom of her composite is written: **"Dad, I Love you."**

Next to the composite is a more current photograph of Kim sitting on a sandy beach enclosed in a large heart that she had traced in the sand.

The picture frame containing her photo has the writing: **"Dad, you set an example I'll follow for life. To do what is right, to try my best, to show respect, your words ring true in my head and heart. Thanks for being my teacher and my best friend, Dad."**

Next to Kim's photos and composite is a picture frame with a message enclosed from Ardith, which says, in part: ***"To My Husband—You are the most important person in my life and I want you to know I'm happy and proud to be your wife...***

You leave an indescribable void during even the shortest of separations... You are a special man and I'm thankful God gave you to me, for you are not just my husband, but my friend and favorite company."

Whenever I look at these messages from my entire family, it makes me feel really good inside, knowing that this truly represents my wonderful and loving family.

The love that flowed toward me simply made me want to do more than ever for my family. As far as I am concerned, nothing was ever too good for my family, and there is nothing that I would not do for them, if I could.

On the following pages are some of the plaques my wife and daughters gave me that I continue to proudly display. I will always love them and cherish their plaques.

To My Husband

You are the most important
person in my life
And I want you to know I'm
happy and proud to be your wife

We don't always agree on everything
there are times you are an exasperation
But you leave an indescribable void
during even the shortest of separations

You have been a loving husband
if not always the most serene
A man who makes his presence felt and
whose family holds in high esteem

You have a great sense of humor
which is such a marvelous trait
You can make people laugh and
cause tense situations to dissipate

You are a special man and
I'm thankful God gave you to me
For you are not just my husband
but my friend and favorite company

Ardith

Cathy

He's My Hero

My hero is the one I walk with.
My hero is the one I talk with.
My hero is always by my side.
My hero's tummy is kind of wide.
My hero is always there for me.
My hero makes me always to see.
My hero is there to pick me up
when I'm down.
My hero never lets me frown.
My hero is thoughtful and kind.
My hero thinks of me all the time.
My hero fixes my car when its on
the wack.
My hero also cracks my back.
My hero is great, its me who's proud.
My hero can also get quite loud.
My hero is the best chiropractor around.
My hero is always to be found.
My hero is my dad, I'm glad to say.
I'm sure he's yours now from day to day.

Cathy 80

Kim

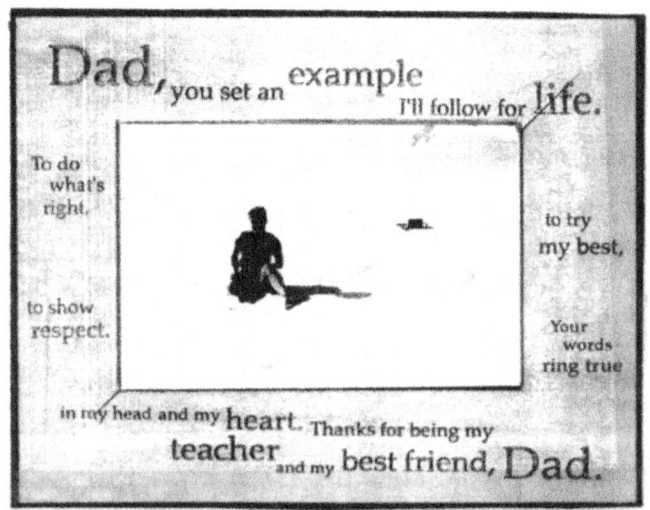

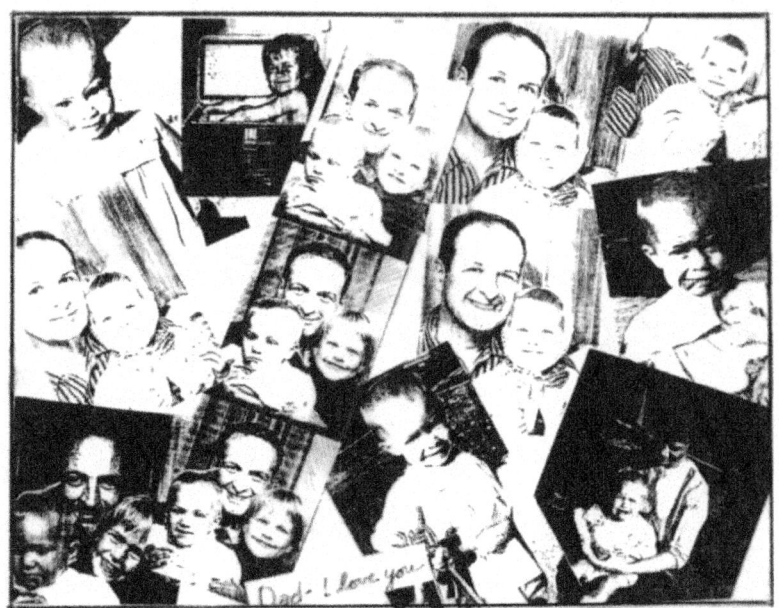

Cindy

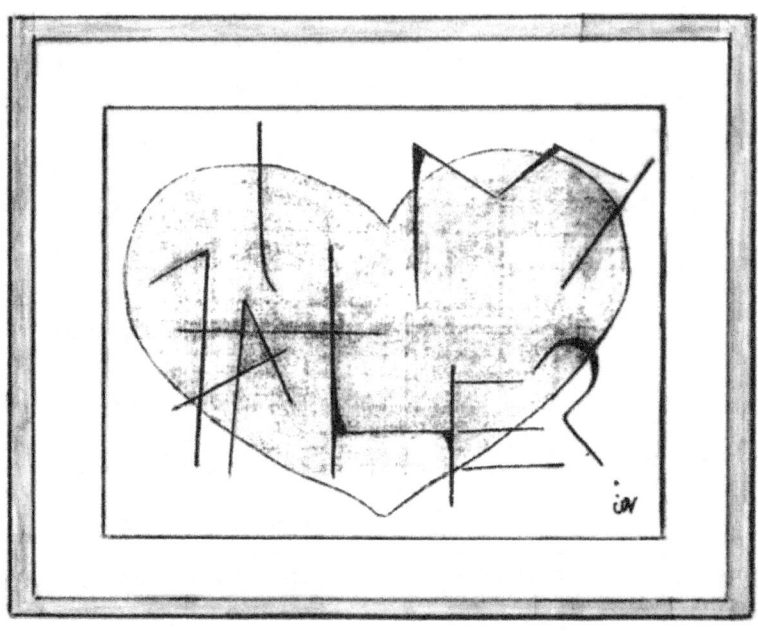

To Dad-
Happy Father's
Day! Thanks for being
supportive over the past
few years. You're the greatest-
I mean it.
Love
Cindy your
son daughter
1997

Even though I have received many recognition plaques and awards throughout my long-time career, I would not trade even one of the plaques given to me by my wife and daughters for all of the others.

I felt guided and protected by Christ. I shared my firm belief with my wife, Ardith, and my daughters. I insisted that I had been chosen to make a difference in healthcare. My family members mistakenly perceived this as delusions of grandeur, but I simply stated it as an upcoming event.

My wife left me and all three of my daughter turned against me. I would much rather have my family back and remain unknown, but this was not in God's plan, and so, as Rev. David Jeremiah says, ***"If you are going to brag on anyone, brag on Christ."***

As I sat at my computer, I would tell Ardith how I had asked Christ to guide me in my writings, and that I had been given the responsibility of correcting the dishonest conduct of the American Medical Association. Ardith did not believe me, and would say, "Oh, why would God use you if you don't even go to church, and when you do, you fall asleep?"

Christ initially faced a similar problem of acceptance from his immediate family. He noted that a prophet is not without dishonor, except within his own house. The only answer I could come up with at that time was that my guidance had to come from God.

I learned later, after reading the Bible, that we are all sinners and that Christ used a murderer, zealot, and a corrupt tax collector, and that I was not that good, but because I made some serious mistakes in my early days, which would be used later to fulfill a special mission for Christ.

Instead of Ardith believing me, she insisted that I loved chiropractic more than I loved her, which was a malicious lie straight from hell. I told her that she was the most important person in my life. She said that since I loved chiropractic more than her, she put our children ahead of me after Christ.

Ardith should have known better, but the devil had her convinced. I told Ardith that I loved her very much, but I hated how the over-utilization of drugs and surgery were causing **thousands of unnecessary deaths and suffering every week!**

This is what motivated me to act, and not my love for chiropractic. It was six years later and I was still trying to win her back to me. So, that's not love?

I felt a compelling hatred toward the policies of the AMA, which were similar to those used by the Nazi's during WWII, while 3,000 people were dying every week because of public ignorance about what constituted rational and safe healthcare, while chiropractic, which could prevent some of these unnecessary deaths, was under attack.

This evil could not go unchallenged, and God gave me the ability to fight it. It was something that I had to do. I explained this to Ardith many times.

It is good for Christians to hate evil, and I hated the AMA's policy of elimination with a passion. I thought, as a professed Christian, Ardith would understand this.

There was no way I could remain silent as these atrocities were happening. These deaths are well confirmed in all of the medical journals; I was not making them up. The medical profession acknowledges them. Chiropractic healthcare could reduce some of these unnecessary tragedies through closer inter-professional cooperation, and yet the AMA was trying to destroy chiropractic.

What was happening was outright obscene. The AMA had to be challenged.

* * *

Ardith decided that she wanted to renew our marriage vows in a small church in Elizabeth, Illinois. It was an emotional experience for me; renewing our vows, especially when I had all three of my daughters, my only granddaughter, Emily, my two sons-in-law, and my favorite adopted niece and nephew all attending.

It was a very special day for me, which I shall never forget.

Whenever I went over to my daughter Cathy's home, who lives only two blocks away, I would immediately walk over to my granddaughter, Emily, and throw my arms around her and give her a great big loving hug, and then swing her around 360 degrees, calling it "an official greeting." When Emily's friends were present and saw this, they wanted the same hug from me, and I took turns hugging and swinging all of them. Emily enjoyed it tremendously whenever Grandpa came over, and she always had a big smile for me from ear-to-ear, waiting for the inevitable hug, and I never neglected giving Emily my official loving greeting if she was present.

I bought a summer home at Apple Canyon Lake for my daughters to enjoy and I planned to gradually divest myself of the property and give it to them. It was spacious and large enough, on two lots, to hold a football field. It was the most beautiful property on the entire lake. We used a golf cart to drive to our pier in front of our home and to the trails and the Association golf course nearby.

Cathy felt that a large deck boat would be a great addition to their summer home and that it would add a new dimension of fun to their weekends. So, I sold my favorite bass boat and helped my daughter purchase a beautiful new deck boat, which could carry 12 to 15 passengers, travel 45 miles an hour for water skiing, and it made a great party boat.

I never cared for the deck boat, as it was too large, so I bought myself a paddleboat for fishing. My family's enjoyment of the summer home meant more to me than my bass boat. I always put my family's interest first, which is what my parents did for me, and so I chose to continue the same policy of giving with my family. My mom and dad were not wealthy, but they were very generous and giving people. They were immigrants from Poland, and all they asked was to work hard and to be able to support their family. They were among the many immigrants of that era who came over and helped make America strong and prosperous.

My parents lived in the back of their Mom and Pop grocery store and worked 15 hours a day, 7 days a week. My dad also worked as a painter. My dad would come home from work and tend to the grocery store as my mother prepared supper. My job was to wash the dishes, circulate the grocery fliers every week throughout the neighborhood, and stack the shelves with new merchandise as it came in. We did this for 11 years.

My parents helped me with my college tuition so that when I graduated I had no school debts. Upon graduation from college, I was drafted into military service and my parents gave me their new automobile so that I could travel about in style and comfort, while most servicemen walked or stayed in their barracks.

My car provided me with a great social life. I went to many dances and met a lot of young ladies. I felt like a spoiled brat while stationed at Fort Lewis, Washington, and deeply appreciated what my parents had done to help make my military life so very pleasant and enjoyable. It was just like an internship working in physical therapy. I even had my fishing tackle and outboard motor in the trunk of my car so that I could fish in the local lakes.

After my discharge from the military, my parents financed me so that I could afford to open my chiropractic office. I told my dad that I would never be able to repay him for what he and Mom had done for me, but I promised him that I would do the same thing for his grandchildren.

In keeping my promise to my dad, I helped all three of my daughters with down payments on their homes, bought them cars, helped them with their school tuitions, and was always available to them whenever they needed any financial assistance.

It got to the point where Ardith would ask, **"Chet, do you suppose we could...?"**

And before she'd finish her question, I would say, **"Okay, to whom and how much?"**

Nothing was too good for my wife and daughters. I was now giving back to my family for the great life that I had enjoyed, because of the loving help I had received from my hardworking, generous, and giving parents.

My daughter, Kim, lived at home during the first two years that she attended a local community college, so I was able to afford to pay for her entire four years of college and buy her a brand new Skyhawk automobile when she went away to college for her last two years.

She eventually moved to Colorado to live in the mountains, and so I bought her a truck as well as a Jeep, and helped her make the down payment on a new home and make some major landscaping improvements as well.

My daughter Cathy had moved to three different homes, and three different times I helped her financially with her homes.

I even took out a large mortgage on my own home to help her purchase a house two blocks away, so that she could live close to Ardith. I also contributed to all kinds of major improvements to Cathy's three homes, including purchasing Paver bricks for her last home.

In the meantime, I helped my daughter Cindy with her first two years of college tuition, with the purchase of a home, and then I gave her significant financial assistance to help her adopt children, because she wanted to be a mother, but was unable to become pregnant.

As a stay-at-home-mom, Ardith had some event going on with our daughters nearly every day, including Girl Scout activities, cheerleading, and soccer games. You might say that we were an All-American model family, yet it seemed that the more Ardith and I did for our girls, the more demanding and less appreciative they became, and gradually they became disrespectful. It was a very gradual decline beginning in the early 2000s.

One day, Cindy flew into a vicious verbal attack against me. Nobody understood why. It was later learned that she had grossly perverted some facts, and an apology would have been appropriate from her, but I never received that apology. When I would bring it up, Ardith would say, "Oh, just let it go. Forget it. It's not that important anyway."

But Cindy's unbridled insults became worse and more frequent. If I had done the same thing to Cindy, my wife would have been all over me to apologize. There was definitely a double standard.

Over time, Cindy's attitude began to negatively influence her sisters, and all three girls were gradually becoming less and less respectful towards Ardith and me.

Cindy told her mother that she hated me for the past five years because I did not pay for her last two years of college. When I asked Ardith if Cindy was justified in such hatred, Ardith replied that she did not know. She was too intimidated by Cindy to take a stand.

Despite all I had done for her and all the love I had for her, Cindy showed Ardith and me nothing but disrespect. The devil was slowing gaining ground.

After Cindy graduated from college, I gave her money to purchase a home. She told me I was the greatest father in the world. Later, when she found out she could not bear children, I gave her money to help adopt children. I believe her inability to conceive was due to the stress and hatred that she harbored.

I did not pay for Cindy's last years of college because she had squandered the college funds that I had given her. I had a drawer full of parking tickets from the time she lived in the Lincoln Park area, but no apologies. Unless you had a garage in the Lincoln Park Area, there are very few legal parking places on the street. Cindy could have easily lived at home, gone to college downtown, and not had dozens of parking tickets, plus she could have saved money by not having to pay for the extra high rental she was paying at Lincoln Park. I felt it was time Cindy learned to take responsibility for her actions, so I did not pay for her last two years of college.

When I had tried to reason with her during that time, she would yell, *"La, La, La, La, I can't hear you!"*

Why she was bringing up ancient history years later, like my refusing to pay her last years of college tuition, puzzled and saddened me. I was completely shocked. I could not believe this was happening.

Ardith's typical reaction to our daughters' voicing criticism or showing disrespect to us was, *"Oh, just forget it. Let it be. It's not that important anyway."*

Unbridled and unchecked, the disrespectful instances gradually became more and more frequent.

When John was out of work or when my granddaughter Emily needed extra money for special tutoring, I was there for them with the money. Cathy and her family got to use our summer home for nine years and never had to pay one penny toward real estate taxes, insurance, Association fees, repairs, or utilities. They had a golf cart and a new boat at the summer home, which they could ride to the pier in front of the house, and they could drive the cart to the Association golf course for golfing.

They were living like millionaires, and yet it was becoming apparent that all the love that had been shared through the years was very gradually degenerating, and becoming judgmental and disrespectful. I saw this as ingratitude on their part, because Ardith and I had done many things for them through the years.

A couple of years earlier, I was told I was the greatest father and husband in the entire world, yet gradually during our last year of marriage, my daughters' and my son-in-law's affection for me was taking a gradual decline for no valid reason.

It is extremely painful and difficult for me to write about my family in this book, because I love all of them very much and do not want to hurt them. I want to strongly re-emphasize here that this is NOT about my wife and daughters' conduct, but about how the devil was able to manipulate himself into my family. The devil can manipulate the best of families, if you allow it to happen. No one is exempted—not even my family—all of whom are good people.

God is not just using me, he is using the entire Wilk family as an example, and hopefully Ardith will recognize this and will join with me in this battle to save our daughters. It has been over six years since our divorce and I have not given up on my family, nor will I ever.

As time went by, it seemed that my family interactions were becoming more challenging and more negative. There was never a big explosion or confrontation of any kind, and yet the wonderful relationships I had with my wife and daughters began to erode little by little.

I never expected to lose them, but the devil had other plans for me.

* * *

Ardith had offered to pay for Cathy's tuition to become a beautician, since Cathy had chosen to not attend college, but she was getting sick from working around hair sprays and I was concerned about her health.

Ardith said, "Oh, just give her the money or she'll get mad." I responded, "Why should she get mad? We helped her with all three of her homes. We put our home into a mortgage and gave her the money so that she could live two blocks away, and we bought her a summer home, which she uses without any cost to her."

Cathy came over for the money and Ardith told her, **"Dad wants to talk with you first."**

Cathy, sensing Ardith's apprehensiveness, made a rude remark about where she would not kiss me for the money, and then she walked out. She then called her sister Cindy, who telephoned me. Cindy went into an angry tirade against me.

Cathy then called and added to Cindy's attack by saying, "Mom, you should have told Dad to give you the money or you would pack up and move out!"

Ardith became hysterical and said, **"I guess we old people just have to die and get out of their way."**

Cathy was in her 30s at that time and had already received all kinds of financial assistance from me, and certainly had no such entitlement. Cathy was totally out of line, but Ardith, afraid of losing Cathy, would not stand up to her.

The next morning, Ardith flew out to California to be with Cindy for one week. Five days later, Ardith called me on the telephone and said she was not returning home and wanted a divorce. There were no harsh words spoken between Ardith and me. All of the anger and hostility was coming from my daughters. I was completely shocked. I could not believe this was happening.

* * *

I truly believe that Ardith developed Stockholm Syndrome while living with Cindy, who constantly and adamantly opposed any reconciliation attempts between her mother and me.

An estimated 15 percent of the population can succumb to the Stockholm Syndrome, if exposed to the following threatening situations:

1. **A perceived threat to survival and belief that the captors will make good their threats.** Ardith felt our daughters would abandon her if she came back to me, and losing her daughters was a fate worse than death in Ardith's mind.

2. **Perception of small kindnesses from the captors within an atmosphere of terror.** While in California, Ardith said over the phone, *"Oh Chet, you should see how loving everyone is to me!"* But within this so-called *loving environment,* Ardith believed that if she returned to me, our daughters would become hostile towards her and disown her as their mother.

3. **Isolation from outside views other than those of the captors.** Ardith was sequestered in California. My phone calls were not returned and my letters were returned marked *"refused,"* with nasty writings on them in Cindy's handwriting.

4. **Perceived inability to escape.** Ardith saw no escape. If she returned to me, she would lose the love of her daughters.

Psychologists say that it takes three to five days to create the Stockholm Syndrome in a victim. On the fifth day of her California stay with Cindy, Ardith asked me for a divorce. Five days with Cindy, and Ardith went from, **"I guess they want us old people to die and get out of their way"** to **"I want a divorce."**

* * *

Whenever I gave my daughters money to purchase a home, I reserved the right to agree that their choice of property was a good investment.

Kim had wanted to purchase a house that she could not live in as a firefighter, because it was too far away from the fire station. Giving her the money would have been like putting a noose around her neck, as it would have been a large mortgage for a home she would not be able to live in.

I refused to give her money that would only put her into a serious predicament. I did not see this purchase as a wise choice.

Cathy had wanted to purchase a house that was a 100-year-old, "teardown" frame shack in a bad neighborhood. I told her the building was a disaster, and her husband, John, agreed.

I insisted that the real estate had to be a good investment before I was willing to give my daughters money to purchase property, and so they labeled me as being "controlling and manipulative." They did not have to return the money I gave them, but I had to feel good about giving them money to purchase a decent property.

Ardith would only say, **"Oh, just give them the money and let them fall on their faces with it!"**

I disagreed and felt that was a terrible and mean thing to say! You don't give money to deliberately hurt people and have them fall on their faces with it. I could not hurt my daughters in that way. This was the devil talking.

All of my daughters eventually bought nice homes with my help, but their irrational belief that I was **"controlling and manipulating them"** remained.

The devil was winning.

Cindy had parlayed her financial gift from me into two condos and a beautiful home, and was initially very grateful for my help, but a couple of years later, reversed her opinion of me for no apparent reason. At the time, I did not understand, but then I didn't know much about Jesus or about the devil's ways yet. I later read the Bible and then it became very clear—it was the devil's work.

I often complimented Cindy on her entrepreneurial genius and ability as a special education teacher. Her negative attitude towards me could only be coming from the devil.

One time when Cindy was very young, perhaps eight years of age, she kept repeating out loud to herself, *"I foiled him. I foiled him. I foiled him!"*

Others heard what she was saying and asked, *"Whom did you foil?"*

She responded, *"I foiled the devil! He wanted me to do it, but I foiled him."*

Everyone laughed and thought it was very cute coming from a small child, but looking back, could it have been the devil testing Cindy? As I look back, it seems that this incident was a foreshadowing of things to come.

I retained three different independent Christian marriage counselors and received extensive counseling from each of them. I wanted to understand if I was truly the one responsible for my wife leaving and my daughters acting hostile towards me.

All three counselors concluded that my daughters were spoiled and outrageously unreasonable. I offered to pay for their counseling sessions if they would consult with my counselors, even if they did it by phone, but all three of my daughters refused, insisting that they didn't need counseling.

Ardith, who was living over 2,000 miles away, also still rejected my marriage counseling offers.

One of my counselors became so thoroughly disgusted with my family's conduct, that she said, *"Dump them! They aren't worth it."*

The devil even got to one of my counselors. The devil was very much in control.

After my divorce from Ardith was final, Cathy called me at 1:30 in the morning, crying that she missed me, loved me, and wanted to resume our father-daughter relationship. I was pleasantly surprised by her call and responded, "That's great! Let's talk to Mom about getting back together again."

When I said this, Cathy became enraged, insisting that I was **using her as a pawn to get her mother to return to me.** She rejected any further reconciliation.

She had initially told her mother to pack up and leave me, and now wanted to keep her own mother out of any family reunion. Still, when confronted, Cathy insisted that she played no role in our divorce whatsoever and that children were **never** the cause of divorce.

After our divorce, Ardith sent me a carefully handwritten 8-page letter explaining why she left me. It was a sweet and kind letter, but she was thoroughly confused. I prepared a reply to her letter.

In fact, there were no harsh words spoken between Ardith and me. The only harsh words came from our daughters. I was more than generous to everyone, and Ardith acknowledged my generosity in her letter. So why leave me?

Eleven times in her 8-page letter, Ardith repeated that she felt **"unloved."** I told Ardith on many different occasions during our marriage that I loved her very much, that she was the most important person in my life, and that I would be lost without her, and I meant every word of it. It was over two years later, and I was still trying to win her back. The devil had Ardith convinced of a lie.

My hatred toward the AMA's attempts to destroy my profession while thousands of people were dying every week from **unnecessary** medication and surgery had prompted me to give a lot of attention to the lawsuit. Putting so much time and effort into the lawsuit, along with working in my practice made me preoccupied at times and required me to travel at times, but I loved Ardith and I thought she understood how much, and also how important the lawsuit was to me. It meant saving thousands of lives in the long run.

I now believe that while I was focused on saving lives, the devil was focused on convincing Ardith that I did not love her.

The devil had obviously blocked Ardith's memory. She was a victim of the devil and did not realize it.

I responded to Ardith's letter and stapled my response to her letter. When she came over to pick up her belongings, I handed it to her in front of our home. Cathy grabbed both letters from Ardith, threw them on the ground, and said, ***"No!"***

This was a vicious attack by Cathy against both her mother and me. Ardith sheepishly went to Cathy's car, sat down in the front seat, and didn't say a word. I picked the letters up from the ground and handed them to Ardith again. Cathy reached up and grabbed the letters from Ardith again, threw them out of the window, then got into her car and they drove away.

A few minutes later, Ardith ran back on foot, all winded from running, since Cathy lived two blocks away, and passionately defended her daughters as being "good girls," and said that she loved me, but that she couldn't live with me.

My adopted niece and nephew were present and witnessed the entire incredible event.

Afterwards, Cathy acknowledged that she had done wrong by grabbing my letters from her mother, but the devil had her believe that it was only done on an ***"impulse."*** Cathy's so-called innocent impulse was the devil using deceit and compulsion on her. Cathy was in a spiritual battle with the devil and needed to ask Christ to guide and help her.

This was Satan at his best using every devious trick in his book against Cathy.

Cathy did not let me see my granddaughter Emily, and Emily, being a youngster, could not understand why her Grandpa wasn't coming over to see her. Emily would ask, "Why doesn't Grandpa come over? Doesn't he love me anymore?"

The love Emily had for Grandpa was stolen from her and replaced with sadness. And where was Ardith on this tragedy? Totally unaware of how her granddaughter was hurt in the process.

This is truly heartbreaking to me.

Cathy wanted to resume a loving father-daughter relationship with me, but did not want Ardith and me to reconcile as husband and wife! This was a divisive attack on both her mother and father.

I wrote kind, conciliatory, and loving Christian letters to Cathy, telling her that she needed to find Christ and that she was a victim of the devil. Christ said, ***"Blessed are the peacemakers for they shall be Sons of God."*** My letters were not hostile or threatening. I urged her to speak with my counselor and told her that I'd pay for it.

Cathy resented my letters and responded with hateful, angry, and sarcastic words.

Then it got even uglier as the devil was fighting back.

Cathy actually took me to court, insisting that I was harassing her with my letters. I urged Cook County's Judge Thaddeus Machnik, who was not a Christian, <u>to read my letters,</u> and he said, "Toohy" (As if he was spitting), saying he would not read the letters as they were "personal." Without reading my letter, he put a restraining order on me without even understanding the truth of what had been taking place.

I was not allowed to contact Cathy or my granddaughter. Satan had influenced the judge.

Any cursory read of my letters would have shown the judge that he'd made a reckless and huge mistake with his restraining order, and that he hurt an innocent child, my granddaughter, in the process.

* * *

I felt that it was time to start contacting all of the 50 State chiropractic organizations and, once again, become active with chiropractic, while also bringing chiropractors to Christ and exposing the devil's role in healthcare.

I spent the past two years trying to persuade Ardith to return to me without success. Neither my wife nor my three daughters had any contact with me. Still, I felt that all these crazy things were happening for a reason, and that somehow it would be corrected.

After contacting all 50 State chiropractic associations, the first chiropractor to contact me was Dr. Timothy Gay, a prominent chiropractor from San Diego. After confirming a speaking engagement, I casually mentioned that my ex-wife resided in the San Diego area. Dr. Gay asked me what town Ardith lived in and I told him that it was in Encinitas.

Dr. Gay responded, "I live in Encinitas! Where about does she live?"

I gave him her address and he said he knew exactly where Ardith lived and that it was about one mile from his home. I was astounded! What were the odds that the first doctor to make an appointment for me to speak lived within a mile of Ardith?

The United States covers about 3.8 million square miles. This means that the odds of this happening were nearly one in four million.

But the incredible events did not stop there. Dr. Gay had the **exact same last name** as a Dr. Gay who had been a former senior minister at my church years earlier and, in fact, he was the minister that had counseled Ardith and me in the past. This was incredible! I would be speaking virtually at Ardith's doorstep.

I was absolutely convinced that this had to be God setting this up, so I sent Ardith a note telling her what had happened and where and when I would be speaking, and she was invited, but she never showed up.

I believed that God was on our side, trying to get us back together to mend our marriage. **(Pastor Gay was NOT the same minister who refused to tell Ardith to get marriage counseling.)**

Questions We Need to Ask.

Why did Cathy tell her mother to pack up and leave me, and then insist that she played no role in the divorce of her parents?

How could Cathy insist that children were **never** the cause of divorce, when she clearly influenced her mother into divorcing me after many, many years of marriage?

Why did Cathy call and tell me she loved me and wanted to renew our relationship, but withdrew her offer to reunite after I asked her to speak with her mother about reuniting as a family? Why did she want to keep her very own mother out of her family reunion loop?

Why did my daughter Cindy resurrect an old irrational hatred from college days, when she had expressed her love, praise, and affection for me after college?

Why did my daughter Kim tell me that she never wanted to have anything to do with me ever again because I put hot water in her mother's coffee to reduce her caffeine intake? And she gave no other reason. Why did Ardith abandon me for no reason other than feeling *"unloved,"* after I told her many times that she was the most important person in my life?

Why did she hire a non-Christian lawyer, flee to California, refuse Christian marriage counseling, and file for divorce? Why did she insist on renewing our marriage vows and then cavalierly violate her marriage vows before Christ for a second time—and for absolutely no logical reason? The answer to all of these questions is the same— it was the devil's influence. He was very much in control.

The Rest of the Story.

Ardith was not a disciplinarian and allowed her daughters to get away with disobeying and being disrespectful to us, their parents, without suffering any punishment or consequences. Ardith was easily manipulated and would not stand up to our girls.

There was virtually no discipline in our home; the kids ran the home more than Ardith. Ardith said that she and her brother never got a spanking in their entire lives. Ironically, she has had no communication with her brother for over 40 years, a brother whom she said she loved so dearly. This is the devil's work.

Ardith uncompromisingly insisted that spanking was cruel and wrong and that the girls would get better as they got older. No marriage counselor will agree with Ardith on that point.

The Bible teaches that discipline needs to be started at an early age. If it is done unilaterally, the person doing the disciplining becomes the villain, and this only makes matters worse and sends the wrong message.

Focus on the Family advocates spanking, **but with love and not with anger,** and the kids need to know that spanking is being done for their own good.

I tried spanking when frustrated and angry, which sent the wrong message, especially when the girls knew their mother was totally opposed to any kind of spanking. They knew that we were divided on this issue.

Today, kids are locked into special seats with seatbelts in their cars, but when the Wilk family would travel, the three girls would often became very boisterous and even wrestle in the car while it was in motion, which created very hazardous driving conditions, while Ardith refused to have them settle down in their seats and behave themselves. Today, drivers could get fined for allowing this kind of conduct in cars.

I respected Ardith's Christian stand through the years, but said that I'd leave the spiritual part up to her while I focused on the secular part. This was very wrong on my part. I was convinced that I was chosen by Christ for a special mission, but my daughters did not believe me, and perceived it as my being egotistical and delusional.

I would rather have my family saved by Christ more than all the money and fame in the world. I tried to be a good provider, protect my family, remain faithful and true to my wife and daughters, and fulfill my mission in life. Unfortunately, I was ignorant of the Bible, which created serious problems.

After Ardith abandoned me, I was thoroughly devastated. I turned to Christ and began seriously studying the Bible for the first time, and seeing things from a Biblical perspective. I realized how I failed to support Ardith, and made a dreadful mistake by not helping her bring our girls to Christ.

Ardith strongly believed in Christ as her Savior, but she was a pushover and needed a strong Christian partner who supported her. Consequently, our daughters perceived their mother as a religious nut and me as being a non-Christian.

Ardith's mother, who lived with us, insisted that there was no devil, which created another fatal complication. Satan loves people who deny his existence. They become his favorite.

Ardith's mother never had a kind word for anyone and was vocally critical of my lobbying efforts to get chiropractic healthcare included in Medicare for senior citizens. She selfishly insisted that I should ignore helping seniors, and sarcastically called her granddaughters *"Medicare Babies."*

The girls would hear this insult, while Ardith would allow her mother to carry on, saying, *"Oh, just let her talk. She is old and senile."*

I responded with, "Our family members are either too young or too old to behave properly or responsibly, but when will anyone in our family ever reach an age of becoming responsible for their conduct?"

Ardith would laugh at my comment, but there was more tragic truth than humor in my statement. Ardith's mother insisted that we were treating her nicely because of her money—money she would not have had if she had not been living with us free of charge for four years while collecting her social security checks. She was penniless when we took her in, but the devil was able to deceive and convince her of this obvious lie.

If you remove Christ, parental guidance, and discipline from a family, add in a critical mother-in-law who insists there is no devil—and a wife who believed everyone, including innocent babies, will go to hell if not saved—you give Satan the ideal opportunity to enter into the family and manipulate them like a violin. Such was the case with my family.

The Devil Waited for the Right Time to Strike.

The girls were spoiled; they received money and all kinds of material things by simply asking for them. They were given homes, cars, summer homes, and boats, but not brought to Christ, or ever taught to respect and honor their parents! Our errors came back to bite us.

The devil knew that he could not take over the family in the early 2000s with all of these lavish gifts being distributed, but in due time, the girls would become vulnerable.

He had to wait for the right time, but he knew that the girls already had three strikes against them by the way they were raised by Ardith and me, and with the added negative influence of a meddling mother-in-law, it was only a matter of timing for Satan to use his destructive and divisive influence.

If there is anyone who does not believe that the devil has the power to take over and control the minds of people, they are grossly underestimating him. But, he cannot gain entrance unless we allow him to do so. My family left our doors wide open by our conduct.

I learned a harsh lesson and now realize that this is why I was chosen for this role. It was not that I was that good, but because I was that bad, and combined with my wife and mother-in-law, we created a situation that needed to be made public for the entire world to see, so that others could learn from our mistakes.

I believe our experiences will provide a great lesson for other families. In reality, we will be serving Christ in this manner, and we should feel honored to do so.

The Wilk family provided the perfect combination of wrong doings for the devil to really take over and blind, confuse, and control the family. The chemistry was perfect for the devil to enter.

And so, as Paul Harvey would say, "You now have the rest of the story!"

Winning the antitrust lawsuit against the AMA was a major setback for the devil, and he was fighting back by attacking my family with blatant lies. His modus operandi is his lies. He is a master liar.

Christ encourages righteous judgment, but those who took part in the destruction of my family—the Park Ridge minister, the Encinitas, California, counselor, my daughters, my mother-in-law, my wife, the Cook County judge—all have allowed the devil to control them.

* * *

I had a drugless diploma, which I did not display, because it was not necessary, since my chiropractic diploma covered all of my work. My daughter Cathy liked it, so I gave it to her. Satan was able to later convince her to give it away at a yard sale in Chicago instead of returning it to me. This diploma contributed to paying for all three of Cathy's homes, cars, summer home, and boat, all of these years. Only the devil could be so uncaring and unappreciative and control people this way *if we allow it to happen.*

The devil overplayed his hand and it backfired on him in a major way.

The man who bought my diploma recognized my name and called me to see if it had been accidentally thrown away, since people don't discard diplomas while they are still living. I explained to him what happened and he was kind enough to return my diploma to me.

Incredibly, the kind gentleman returning my diploma was named John, the same first name as Cathy's husband, while the maiden name of the mother of the man returning the diploma, amazingly, was "Wilk," the same as Cathy's maiden name! This was surreal. Only God could have done something like this. Wilk is not a common last name; I only found two in the entire Chicago Telephone Directory. This Wilk was not even related to me, as she was Jewish.

The miracle did not stop here.

When John returned my diploma, he brought with him a copy of my earlier book, **Medicine, Monopolies and Malice**, which his mother had purchased 15 years earlier, and had it completely highlighted. Her son said that she had read it thoroughly. For her to have purchased my book out of almost 300 million people in America was in itself one chance in a 100,000. This was Divine Guidance. John had me autograph his mother's copy.

Combine this amazing story of my book and diploma with the fact that a couple of years earlier, I was asked to speak to a group of chiropractors, by Dr. Timothy Gay, who lived over 2,000 miles away, but within one mile of Ardith. Dr Gay had the **exact same last name** as the minister at my Park Ridge Church, who actually counseled Ardith and me.

This was Divine Intervention! This kind of information cannot be fabricated. As unbelievable as it is, it is very easily verifiable.

If I held one ounce of bitterness towards my family because of their outrageous conduct, the devil would grin and say, "I gotcha!" And he will have won the battle. Instead, he lost the battle big time and was clearly exposed in the process.

If both parties in a marriage understood the devil's modus operandi, the divorce rate would be greatly reduced and we'd have happier marriages. I believe this book will help many families recognize how the devil works. **We need to attack the devil and not blame our spouses.**

If we know whom our real enemy is and are appropriately prepared for him, we have a better chance of avoiding being bushwhacked by him.

The devil has tried everything he can to stop this book from being published by attacking my family. I see this as spiritual warfare, and I believe this book will be read by millions of people and it will open their eyes to the truth that not only is there is a God in heaven, but that there is a devil in hell. Besides dividing and undermining health care and getting into politics, the devil also gets into the judicial system. We have witnessed it with a judge who refused to read my letters and put an injunction on me because I was trying to save my marriage.

It is the same judicial system that supports removing God from schools and public places. It's the same judicial system that puts drunk drivers in jail for killing people, but supports medical doctors getting paid for killing innocent children.

Last, but not least, this book exposes the devil for dividing families. You can see the plaques and love that emanated from my family, and the sentiments were genuine until the devil stepped in and took over.

My daughters are solid citizens whom any father would be very proud of, but they are victims of the devil. Hating me for adding hot water to my wife's coffee, or for not paying the last two years of college tuition, or because I was concerned about my daughter working around hair sprays because of her allergies, is pathological behavior that can only come from the devil.

The devil represents hate, whereas God loves us not by what we do and what we are, but ***in spite of what we do and what we are! This is the unconditional and agape love that I have for my family.***

Ardith and my divorce should be viewed as a tragedy that will be turned into a victory over the devil, because it prompted the writing of this book.

God knew this book would be written before I was born, and Christ guided its writing. I'll explain what I mean at the very end of the book. You will be amazed.

And for Attorney McAndrews to have been put into the time and place to do what no other attorney could have—or would have done—was God's work. This was no coincidence.

With the facts that are presented in this book, it would be sheer insanity for anyone to try to raise a family in our corrupt society without using the Bible for guidance. Every family needs exposure to Christ on a daily basis, and not just on Sundays.

People would not consider eating meals one day a week to nourish their bodies any more than they can expect to nourish their souls by coming to Christ one day a week.

Living for Christ needs to be a 24-hour, 7-day-a-week commitment.

Christ already defeated Satan on the cross when He saved us from Satan's bondage. Satan is responsible for causing many problems everywhere, yet escapes being exposed as the real culprit. This is the way he operates, and he has thousands of years of experience in how to deceive people.

We are in a major spiritual warfare and he wants to devour us. Nobody can outsmart the devil alone without accepting Christ as their Savior, asking for His grace, and having Christ guide them.

When a minister violates the Bible and refuses to face up to his wrongdoings, and stonewalls anyone who calls attention to his inappropriate conduct, it shows just how deceptive and influential the devil can be. But in the eyes of God, they are the biggest hypocrites.

Christ is the only way to win the spiritual battle that we all face.

* * *

Chapter 5

Conclusive Evidence—The Devil is Real

The following pages will provide absolute proof beyond all reasonable doubt that there is a God in heaven and a devil in hell. If you are a Christian, you will acknowledge that what I have experienced is the work of God, and that there is indeed a devil.

If you are a nonbeliever, you will not be able to stand up to the evidence, which I present here. I am not an expert on the Bible by any stretch of imagination, but no one can stand up to the conclusive evidence that I have provided in this last chapter. If you try to defend your position, YOU will lose big time! It will be no contest. The facts are so solid.

Most people believe that there are guardian angels, and some even provide their personal experiences as proof. Pope Benedict XVI said that his guardian angel was clearly acting on "superior orders" when he let him fall and fracture his wrist so that it would teach him more patience and humility, and give him more time for prayer and meditation.

When I was a child, we had a family friend, by the name of Mrs. Budek, who came to my home to visit periodically over a 15-year period. She always came over unannounced and would tell me exactly what I would be doing in the future. She was never wrong.

She made over 20 different predictions about my

future and what I'd be doing in fine detail, and every one of them came out 100 percent exactly as she said. I had two different perceptions of her, but I was wrong in both cases. And then I read this old news item of how Pope Benedict fractured his wrist and for the first time, I realized what I had been missing for over 70 years! Mrs. Budek was my guardian angel! She was very protective of my family and me, and in one instance, probably even saved my life. Amazingly, it took a Pontiff's fractured wrist to make me see the truth.

Why was Christ using this guardian angel to guide me all of these years? What could be Christ's motive? God doesn't do things without a reason. The only answer that I could come up with was so that I could write this book and inform people about God from firsthand experience, and to tell them that there is a devil. Everyone will have to agree that fulfilling 23 predictions with 100 percent accuracy is supernatural, that it exceeds all statistical probabilities, and that it has to come from God. There is no other logical explanation.

Meanwhile, the devil could never support a book like this because he would be attacking himself, and Christ even said that the devil could never attack himself and survive.

As I reflect back at what has happened in my life, the devil was actually attacking my family and me, and was trying every devious tactic to discredit me and stop this book from coming out for the world to read. We were in a major spiritual battle.

For the benefit of those who may think I am fabricating this story, I took and passed the latest state-of-the-art polygraph test to prove that everything in this book is 100 percent accurate and that nothing has been falsified.

If you are not familiar with what a polygraph test does, an examiner attaches all kinds of instruments to your body and monitors your perspiration, pulse, blood pressure, skin resistance, sweat gland activity, respiration, voice sounds, and facial and body movements with video and audio. They ask you questions while all of these instruments are attached to you, while the sound and video are recording your responses. I took and passed this test, proving that everything I am telling you here is true.

The polygraph is recognized as a valid test by the United States Government, the CIA, Secret Service, police departments, and the Better Business Bureau, and that it is a legitimate way of ascertaining the truth (or lies) from a person. I took the test because I could not expect people to believe all of these amazing and unbelievable things happening to my nephew and to me unless we both took polygraph tests and passed them.

If that isn't enough proof, then ask my wife and three daughters. They will have to agree, even if grudgingly, that I speak the truth. In fact, they thought I was being narcissistic and self-centered by speaking so openly about these predictions for so many years, and they are now witnessing some of these events occur in their time. Even my wife doubted me and would say, "Oh, why would God use you, you don't even go to church and when you do you fall asleep." I don't know why. Who can truly know God's reasons for doing anything? I can only tell you that I strongly believe that I am meant to pass on a message of faith and to urge all Christians to pay attention to the many ways the devil is influencing our world today.

Nobody can fool a polygraph test. That's why liars, politicians, and criminals avoid them. Since my nephew and I are neither of the above, we will take and pass any polygraph test anyone requests of us. This being said, please read on.

Mrs. Budek somehow always knew exactly when to come over and make some very timely predictions, which always happened exactly as she said in every detail. My family and I initially all took whatever she said with a grain of salt, until after her foretold events began being fulfilled.

She was genuine and had no vested interest. She was unique in that she never accepted one penny for her service, saying that she would lose her God-given gift if she did. She never commercialized her gift. She avoided people and lived like a recluse. Yet, she visited me periodically over a 15-year period and completely outlined my entire life before it happened! In so doing, she was guiding and protecting me, which is what guardian angels do.

It was as if she was on a mission and knew that she was onto something very special and important. Why else would she have dedicated herself to coming over to my home all of those years and foretelling my future, frequently repeating how I would become "very famous?"

Mrs. Budek was a Christian, and she made her daughter swear on a Bible that she would never tell anyone where she lived, because she didn't want to be bothered by people seeking her gift.

In one instance, Mrs. Budek described a bald and thin man who had a heavyset wife with black hair. She told my mother how many children the couple had, and said that they lived to the south of us.

My mother knew exactly who fit this description, and that it was her brother and his wife and children. Mrs. Budek never met them, so she had no way of knowing these facts. So, how in the world could she know so much about my uncle on my mother's side?

Mrs. Budek urged my mother to visit her brother on the following Sunday afternoon after my father and mother closed our grocery store, and she told my mother to tell her brother that their third-born daughter was very sick and needed to see a doctor immediately.

My mother thought to herself, "How can I tell my brother something like this? There is no way I can do that."

Mrs. Budek insisted. "I know you don't believe me, but if you don't go there and tell them, you will hear about the girl's illness through a friend, by telephone, but by then, it will be too late to save her life."

This is exactly what happened. My family received a phone call from a friend, telling them that the girl in Mrs. Budek's prediction was in a hospital with tuberculosis. My parents visited her in the hospital, but her condition was too advanced and she passed away.

I recall my mother often lamenting how she could have saved her niece's life if she had only spoken up, and this incident left an indelible impression on all of us. After that, whenever Mrs. Budek spoke, we listened.

On one of her unannounced visits, Mrs. Budek told us how two robbers would come into our grocery store. She described how they would look, that they would be wearing Russian fur hats, and warned us that they were extremely dangerous. She strongly admonished us to be very careful and to not do anything foolish because **"they mean business!"**

Soon afterwards, two armed gunmen came into our grocery store wearing Russian fur hats and held us up at gunpoint. As they were leaving, one of them took a bullet out of his gun, placed it into the palm of his hand, showed it to my mother and said, **"I just want to show you that we mean business!"** Once again, Mrs. Budek was trying to protect all of us from injury.

These were the *same exact words* that Mrs. Budek had used. I'll never forget the expression of disbelief on my mother's face when she repeated what the gunman had said to her. She cautioned me about a perilous marine experience. I was fishing one day and the wind picked up suddenly, and I narrowly escaped capsizing the boat. For

94

a while, I didn't know if I would make it. On another of her visits, Mrs. Budek said I would be standing up, vigorously peddling my bicycle, and that I would be approaching an alley that had a garage on either side, creating a blind side. She described the location in exact detail. She said that if I did not heed her warning and slow down, I would be struck by an automobile.

A few days later, I was standing up and vigorously peddling my bike at the location Mrs. Budek had so accurately described. As I approached the alley, I recalled what she had said, so I hit the brake, slowed down, and cautiously entered the alley. As I entered the alley, a car was traveling so fast it seemed like it came out of nowhere, and I ran into the car's running board and was knocked over, but unhurt. I could have been hit broadside and been easily killed had I not slowed down as Mrs. Budek had insisted.

I was in my third semester in optometry school when Mrs. Budek made another of her unannounced periodic visits.

She said, "Chester, you are not going to finish the school that you are in, but a man in a white uniform is going to tell you to leave optometry and follow the same work he does."

She encouraged me to listen to him and change professions. She emphasized I would become "very famous" after switching schools, and that I would make a lot of money. I was not interested in becoming famous or making a lot of money. I just wanted to be a good provider for my family.

Soon after, I went to my uncle to get a chiropractic adjustment for some back pain I was having, and he told me to quit optometry and become a chiropractor like he was. I resisted the idea at first, but I went to the National College of Chiropractic to see if it was my calling, and the rest is history. I became a chiropractor.

When almost finished with Chiropractic College, I was to be drafted into the military, but I was on a deferment. Some of my classmates, who did not go to college, got drafted right out of high school and were killed in action. One of my classmates from high school, Howard Nowotarski, came back from the service with two Purple Hearts.

When my deferment ended, I went into the military. Servicemen were being killed overseas and my mother was understandably concerned. Once again, Mrs. Budek made one of her timely visits and reassured my mother that I would not face any danger, but that I would be going far away and doing something *"like an internship,"* which would be a very good experience. She said that I would be surrounded by large bodies of water.

Mrs. Budek was right again!

I went to Fort Lewis, Washington, and worked in the physical therapy department. It was near the Pacific Ocean, surrounded by the Puget Sound, and, indeed, it was a wonderful experience.

When I opened my office after getting discharged from the military, Mrs. Budek came over and said that I would meet a doctor who would take a great liking to me and that he would be a great help to me professionally.

Shortly thereafter, I met Dr. Amon Hopf, who brought me into his office as an associate. He was a great role model and someone I held in very high regard. I believe that he identified me with his son, Donald, who had passed away, and who would have been my age. He was a unique boy. When people would ask his son if he were going to become a chiropractor like his dad when he grew up, Donald would say, "No, I'm going to be an angel." Donald told his dad to not cry, because he would only be here for a short while.

Robert Swanson, a family friend, can attest to the fact that he heard Donald actually say this. Robert was a pallbearer at Donald's funeral and can confirm this story. Two of Dr. Hopf's dearest and closest friends were Alvin T. Colon, an ordained minister, and his wife, Elvira. When Mrs. Hopf passed away, Dr. Hopf called me and asked me to tell Rev. Colon of her passing.

I called the Colons and relayed the message to Mrs. Colon, who said, "I was in the backyard and I heard what sounded like someone had left the radio on in the house. I came into the house, but the radio was not on; and then I looked over at the piano and there was Mrs. Hopf playing the piano, and she asked me, 'Do you remember that this was the song I played for you the last time I was here?'"

You'll never find a more honest and sincere elderly couple anywhere, and if Mrs. Colon said that she saw Mrs. Hopf playing the piano that afternoon of Mrs. Hopf's death, *prior to my telling her about Mrs. Hopf's death*, removing all possibilities of her hallucinating what she saw. Mrs. Colon would have never fabricated such a story. I would stake my life on it. Rev. Colon said that this was possible and that he had experienced it in the past.

I believe that Christ guided me to meet Dr. Hopf, and arranged to have Dr. Hopf call me so that I could be exposed to Mrs. Colon's supernatural experience, so that I would be able to relay this information to others as solid proof that we all have an eternal soul. It certainly convinced me.

Dr. Hopf retired and I eventually acquired one of the largest chiropractic practices in the City of Chicago.

Mrs. Budek predicted all of these things over 60 years ago. She said that I would be writing books, when it was the farthest thing from my mind. This is now my eighth book.

My nephew, Walter Dziedzic, recalls his mother, my sister, telling him that my wife, Ardith, was going to leave me and that my three daughters would all turn against me, and that I would become "very famous."

My nephew's reaction to my sister's comment at that time was, "No way! How can this be?

His mother went on to say, "It's going to happen. Chester is going to write a book and become very famous."

Walter responded, "But Chester is already famous!" (He was referring to my having sued the AMA and winning a major landmark antitrust lawsuit.)

His mother came back with, "No, he's going to become 'more famous' after he writes a book in which he will add some new information in his book other than chiropractic. You and Chester will become closer, and Chester will become a better Christian."

His mother added, with tears in her eyes, "I wish I could be around so I could say to you, 'See I told you so!'"

Amazingly, Walter's mother died the very next day after telling him this, and Walter will take any polygraph test to confirm that every word here is accurate and true.

I actually recall a rumble many years ago from my sister about how my wife, Ardith, would leave me, but I dismissed it as silly nonsense. At the time, I did not realize that what she was quoting had come from Mrs. Budek.

* * *

My nephew Walter was born a paraplegic, but he could get around very well on crutches. Walter's mother and grandmother often repeated how Walter was going to receive "a lot of money" when he got very old. He grew up hearing about it so many times that he would get irritated by any mention of it.

His response was, "Yah, yah, I know, but I'm 70 years old and I never got any money. I don't believe her."

I reminded Walter about how Mrs. Budek fulfilled other predictions in his family, but he was still unconvinced.

On Thursday, March 24, 2011, I received a phone call from Walter saying that he had been in an automobile accident. His brakes failed in his van and he could not stop. To avoid hitting another vehicle, he veered off the road and into a large tree. He remained conscious long enough to call me on the phone and tell me what happened and which hospital he was in. He sustained multiple fractures of his legs and hips. He spent over a week in intensive care, and then in a nursing home, for a total of about five months. His medical bills were over $600,000.

This brings up another issue as to why medical care should have to cost so much money. It is generally accepted that this is the way it must be, but I strongly disagree. It does NOT have to be. The devil has everyone convinced otherwise.

If Walter had died, then the predictions would not have been fulfilled, but since Mrs. Budek said he would be "getting a lot of money" when he got very old, he would have to survive or she would be wrong for the first time. Even though Walter was in intensive care and the doctors gave him little chance of survival, I had no doubt about him surviving, because his prediction was not yet fulfilled.

Walter finally came home at the end of August. He was nursing an ulcer on the back of his heel. I asked him how this had come about, and he said it was caused by his foot resting on a hard surface while in the hospital. This was very serious. If the infection extended into the bone, his leg might have to be amputated. This was malpractice. Walter contacted a malpractice lawyer and the rest is history. Another prediction was about to be fulfilled.

Nearly two years after the accident, there was still no indication that Walter would ever be able to put weight on his heel. The ulcer still had not healed completely and this was preventing him from putting any weight on his heel without causing pain and further irritating the ulcer.

Being unable to put weight on his foot, he could not exercise to rehabilitate his leg muscles.

Prior to the accident, his muscles had been strong and he was able to walk with crutches, but two years later, he was weaker than ever and required 100 percent nursing care. He could not even get out of bed by himself and had to have his caregiver use a mechanical device with a thoracic harness to lift him out of bed and into his wheelchair. Walter was in great health otherwise, and the doctors said he should live for many years, but he was living in this horrible condition.

There is no doubt that he will receive major compensation for his ulcer, but what a horrific price he has had to pay in order to receive this money. However, it made a believer out of him. All Walter could do was shake his head with disbelief and say, "It's mind boggling!

In spite of all of his hardships, Walter manages to keep his spirits high. I have never heard him complain about his situation. He always has a ready smile for everyone. One day, we were discussing the subject of attitude and how people look at life, and I told Walter how I admired his attitude and that I would not change places with him for all the money in the world. Walter responded by saying that he would not change places with me for all the money in the world, after what I went through by losing my entire family and receiving all of their unjustified hatred, especially after all that I had done to help them.

The Good Lord knows exactly our limits and just how much He can put us through so we can serve Him to the best of our ability.

I was told I would receive both money and fame, while my nephew was told he would receive money, but neither of us were told what a terrible price we would each have to pay in order to receive these. This part was conveniently omitted from Mrs. Budek's predictions, so we could find out for ourselves the grave consequences that would come with it.

The most amazing part is how anyone in this entire world could possibly make such an accurate outline of our lives. We may be the only two people in the world who can say this. It is humanly impossible and defies all logic and common sense—yet it happened and we can prove it with polygraph tests and six individuals to back our facts up.

We had over 20 different predictions fulfilled with 100 percent accuracy in every detail. Just any one of these predictions by themselves was so unique that they individually exceeded all statistical probability. But to have over 20 predictions fulfilled can only come from Divine Intervention. Clearly, God was using my family for a purpose, which was intended for the world to realize that there is a God in heaven and a devil in hell. I believe that what has happened to us will have a major influence on America.

The only possible answer is that it was Divine Intervention and that there had to be a reason for it, since God doesn't do things without a reason. I believe it was so I would write this book and that it would have a major impact on influencing millions of people.

I would rather have the continued love and affection of my family than all the money and fame in the world. However, the Good Lord has other ideas by using my family and me to serve Him.

Walter losing his ability to get around by himself was a priceless and devastating loss, and no amount of money in the world could possibly purchase what he lost on March 24, 2011.

It's all in how we look at life. I see it as God giving me an opportunity to serve Him through my book. It can help millions of other people see the Lord and learn that there IS a devil. History is a great teacher, and this is a history book.

It has been wisely said that to ignore the past is to ignore the future, and to reject the wisdom that it teaches. Perhaps it may even help my family to see the truth. I hope and pray for their sakes that they do. Walter is living proof that we can be as happy as we choose to be. There are many able-bodied people in the world that seem to have everything going for them, yet they do not have the kind of positive attitude Walter has. He can serve as an inspiration for others and remind us of why we should thank God for what we have, since things could always be worse.

I have not revealed all of Mrs. Budek's accurate predictions; I left some of them out for personal reasons, but her involvement in my life made a firm believer out of me that there is a Higher Power, which is God, and that I have been given a special mission in life to use my experience to shine the light for others to see the truth.

If someone is shown more, then more is expected of them. Combined with what I learned from the Bible and from my personal experience, mine is much more than blind faith, but solid, undisputable evidence that proves beyond all reasonable doubt that there is a God in heaven and devil in hell.

If anyone experienced what I have and did not believe in Divine Guidance or Divine Intervention, they would either have to be suffering from major denial and need some serious psychological counseling, or they have no concept of the statistical improbability of foretelling such a large number of events *before* they occurred. It is statistically impossible.

God used my ex-wife, Ardith, to show how a Bible-reading, church-going woman, who reads the Bible for an hour every morning, could change from loving a husband who was true and faithful to her into deserting him and cavalierly violating the Bible without a cause. This is a classic example of the devil's intervention.

It showed how a minister influenced by the devil violated the most sacred obligations of marriages, how my three girls, who loved me and made plaques for me expressing their true love, and then for no valid reasons, all three of them developed a vicious hatred toward me. Within that specific period of time from their 'love to hate,' nothing negative occurred to cause this dramatic change. If you asked them, I doubt they could come up with rational answers. This was the devil's intervention!

My family and I were in spiritual combat, and the devil being a divider, was dividing my family and using hatred as one of his favorite tools.

My daughter, Cindy, openly admitted hating me for five years because I did not pay her last two years of college; my daughter Cathy turned against me because I was trying to restore our marriage, and my daughter Kim said I was too controlling, because I added hot water to my wife, Ardith's, restaurant coffee. These were totally absurd reasons and reveal how the devil uses hatred.

What is even more amazing is that **my guardian angel, Mrs. Budek, predicted that all of these things would happen over 60 years ago!**

By far the most difficult and painful task in writing this book was using my own family to prove that there is a devil. It is NOT an attack on my family as such, but on the devil. And so, the Good Lord provided me with a very talented and dedicated copyeditor in Cheryl Stewart, who helped me to express my thoughts about my family as evidence of the devil's intervention in a clear and gentle way.

As I mentioned earlier, churches and Christian organizations should be devoted to helping the less fortunate members in our society, rather than having our government become a nanny. This should be one of the responsibilities of our churches, but many of our churches have failed us by not even fulfilling their most basic obligation to Christ, which is to unite families with Christ, and not divide them.

Sixty percent of Christians do not believe that the devil is a person, but that he is only a symbol of evil. This clearly shows how our churches have failed to adequately educate its members about the existence of the devil. They need to be more responsible with getting the message out about our enemy. We are in a spiritual war and yet many Christians don't even realize it, or its seriousness. Our battleground is the devil's playground.

Our ministers need to tell it like it is and stop being so condescending or patronizing toward those members who violate Christian principles, and this goes both ways, especially for pastors. Norman Vincent Peale said that the trouble with most of us is that we would rather be ruined by praise than saved by criticism.

Criticism is appropriate, but it must be coupled with a desire to help the other person, or it becomes hypocrisy. Abe Lincoln said, "He has the right to criticize who has the heart to help."

I firmly believe that God knew this book would be written before I was born and guided its writing! If we are given a light, we must shine it for everyone to see and not hide it under a basket.

My divorce from Ardith should be viewed as a tragedy that will be turned into a victory over the devil, because it prompted the writing of this book, and the shining of this light. God allows tragedies to occur so that good can come from them, such as in the case of allowing Christ to be crucified and the ultimate good that came from it to the entire world. I believe this book can save many families from divorce.

America is a very generous and giving nation. After winning the war against Germany, we returned the country back to its people. When we won the war against Japan, we returned the country back to its people.

We did the same thing with Italy. We don't conquer and take over countries; we liberate them.

When removing an evil leader in Iraq, it wasn't to take over the country, but to help rehabilitate the country as a democratic nation and to liberate the people who had been living under the rule of a ruthless dictatorship.

We have been helping other nations in poverty with money, which we don't even have, while our own people are struggling, and yet many of these nations have been ungrateful and hostile to America. **I believe the Good Lord appreciates the generous and giving nature of the American people and is giving us one more chance to save ourselves from our own self-destruction—if we listen! This is one of the main purposes for my book, and I hope President Obama realizes it.**

When hurricane Sandy devastated our East Coast, how many nations came to help us? The answer is none. How many nations came to our help with Katrina? None.

Our nation is on the verge of economic self-destruction and one of its major problems is our healthcare system. It needs a major overhaul before it can be insurable. Nobody can afford to insure it with the unholy alliance that we see between the drug companies and the MD's.

Some of the medical and surgical procedures are outright criminal conduct, and greed, hate, and class envy are the devil's weapons.

Christ said that my people die from a lack of knowledge. While Christ was not specifically referring to healthcare as such, still the obvious lack of knowledge in America can certainly apply to ignorance about what constitutes appropriate or honest healthcare.

Our president needs to do several things, and I believe they came to me as Divine Guidance for President Obama. In fact, if he did these things, he

could still become a hero instead of the president who destroyed our nation!

The president needs to put Obama Care on hold pending a major overhaul of our entire healthcare system. It is killing 3,000 people every week from unnecessary drugs and surgery and the medical journals confirm this fact. It WILL destroy America in its perverted state. Our politicians are arguing over *how to* pay for this perverted and actually fraudulent healthcare system. Our politicians are bickering over a grain of sand as a huge boulder hangs over our heads.

Our legislators should tell the medical profession to straighten out their act. Nobody can insure it the way it is perverted, with its unholy alliance between MD's and the drug industry. Raising taxes will not even scratch the surface of the cost of our overpriced and corrupt healthcare system while the devil has blinded our nation as to what really needs to be corrected.

Healthcare in its present form is not a friendly ally; it has become a lethal adversary. It kills 3,000 people every week. It can bankrupt families with only one major medical catastrophe. In its current state, it is not insurable.

Our healthcare system should be health-oriented, but instead it is disease and symptom-suppression-oriented.

The devil has blinded our politicians and the medical profession by using greed, deception, and class envy as his weapons. We need chiropractors acting as gatekeepers in many of these hospital orthopedic settings. We need more intelligent utilization based on what is in the patient's best interest, not on the drug peddler's or surgeon's selfish economic interests.

In another very serious matter, we need to stop giving money to other countries that literally hate us with a passion. This is outright insanity. We can't buy their

106

love and respect by giving them money that we borrow from China. Only the devil can blind our political leaders to do something that any fifth grade grammar school child should understand. We borrow money that we do not have because we are broke, and then give this borrowed money to hostile countries, who would rather see us annihilated. America can't be a nursemaid for the entire world and be hated for it.

We need to remove the worthless and economically harmful pork barrel spending that is driving us into deeper debt. This is a major problem.

We must retain our military defense as our top priority for freedom. We must never be forced to cut one penny from our defense budget, and, if necessary, we should be able to reinforce it. Our greatest deterrent to war is our military strength.

The last four years we've had no budget, which is **unprecedented, disgraceful, and inexcusable**! This must be corrected. We can't keep spending over a trillion dollars a year more money than we take in. It is suicidal and plays right into the hands of the devil! The United States is the biggest debtor in the world, while China is the biggest military power in the world. Are we going to argue with them if we can't pay them?

Under no circumstances should we ever settle for spending more money than we bring in. There can be no compromise on this issue. The conservative mantra before the election was that America cannot survive four more years of "borrow and spend," and we must mean every word of it! It is MORE than a campaign slogan—it is a FACT! It would be very disingenuous and fatal to stop repeating it now *after* the election. We should repeat it louder and more aggressively than ever so when it happens, we will be able to honestly say, "See, we told you so, but you didn't listen!" Obama will also want to cut our military defense, which will weaken us militarily.

Here is the approach:

"When we said we cannot survive four more years of 'borrow and spend,' we meant every word of it, and that it will destroy our nation unless we wake up to this reality! We don't have a taxing problem but an irresponsible spending problem. Giving our liberal politicians more tax money is like giving drugs to a dope addict or alcohol to a drunk and they will squander more!

The United States has been borrowing 46 cents on every dollar from China just to pay the interest alone, but when our compounded interest exceeds our growth, we will not be able to repay our debt, and we will bankrupt, and don't think for a moment that China will forgive us—look at China's history with human rights. President Obama is playing right into the hands of the devil who hates America and wants to see it destroyed.

Obama's current spending policies will eventually devalue our dollar, cause massive impoverishment, and civil unrest and rioting, unless we wise up before it's too late. Our situation can become worse than in Spain. I hope I won't have to say some day, 'See, I told you so!'"

Are we so naïve that we can't see what is so self-evident? I don't think so. I think this is the work of the devil blinding our nation's leaders so they cannot see the painfully obvious truth. The devil is a divider and hates America because we are a Judeo-Christian nation, and the devil is chipping away at it by using our liberal politicians to remove God from everywhere.

Our country is in a big mess and how we got here is now history. There is enough blame here for virtually everybody to share, whether it be the Federal Reserve, homebuyers, Congress, real estate agents, mortgage brokers, or the Wall Street firms. Most of us have played a role prompted by the devil. The question is: "What can we do now to stop the inevitable from happening?"

President Obama should put Governor Romney on his special advisory committee and listen to what he says, in the nation's best interest. Look at the facts— the best run states in America are blue conservative states, and the worst and most bankrupted are red liberal states. The liberal states are pulling our nation down. What more evidence does anyone need?

It would be a great class act thing to do if the president were to put our nation's welfare ahead of politics. Both political parties should listen to Donald Trump and what he has to offer. We need to listen to the words of experience. He makes a lot of good common sense and he has an unprecedented track record of success unlike anyone else in America. And, by the way, he supported Governor Romney for the presidency. Donald Trump would also make a great president.

If President Obama takes the suggestions outlined above, he still has a chance to save America. He can outwit the devil, who is trying to influence him to destroy our nation, and his positive reversal would impress everyone—conservatives and liberals alike— and his legacy can become as the man who saved America and fixed healthcare.

Most people will say it will never happen, but this is what we MUST do to reverse our current self-destructive path, and the people need to be advised of this _before_ it happens so that when it does, they will realize we are right. If President Obama does not do the right thing, his legacy will most assuredly be as the president who destroyed our great nation.

God is using my entire family and this book as a guide for America to follow. It sounds like a bold and grandiose claim for me to make, but <u>look at the</u> <u>evidence that this book provides!</u> This book is unquestionably being guided by a Divine Power, and has <u>proved itself</u> beyond reasonable doubt!

Have you ever known anyone who experienced 100 percent fulfillment of actually 23 predictions and was never wrong? Is there another human being on earth who can say this and back it up with multiple witnesses and polygraphs as Walter and I can? Fulfilling only one of the predictions is amazing, but fulfilling 23 is supernatural and absolutely impossible from a secular point of view. This took Devine Intervention! And there's more proof.

Let's review a few other examples from previous chapters in this book.

My being invited to speak to an organization by a chiropractor named Dr. Gay, who lives over 2,000 miles away, but also lives one mile from Ardith (one chance in 3.8 million), plus him having the *exact same last name* as the minister in Park Ridge, who counseled Ardith and me, which creates astronomical and impossible odds.

Another example is having my diploma being returned to me (one chance in a 1000) by a man named John (Cathy's husband's name) and his mother's maiden name being Wilk—the exact same last name as Cathy's maiden name (impossible odds), and that John's mother actually purchased my book entitled *Medicine, Monopolies and Malice* 15 years earlier, which means we must multiply all of these impossible odds by another 100,000! These are proven historical facts and cannot be falsified.

With all candor, can anyone with a straight face say that all of these things happening were just luck or coincidental? If so, they are either in serious denial and need psychological help, or they have no concept of their statistical impossibility!

Combine all of these facts with six witnesses, plus my nephew and I willing to take any polygraph test to prove that we speak the truth, and you have a solid case for Christ and against the devil.

Christ guided and protected me, through my guardian angel, by outlining my entire life with 100 percent accuracy, and proved to me beyond all reasonable doubt that God is in charge.

I trust that you have read my book with an open mind. The evidence we have is undeniable and serves to bring some light to the American people during these very troubling times and **what America must do to survive as a nation!**

On the subject of the Bible and the direction that our nation and the world is taking, I strongly urge you to listen to Dr. David Jeremiah on the Internet by simply typing **"Dr. David Jeremiah-Iran Intimidating the world"** into your search engine.

You can see and hear him 24-7. You better be seated when you hear what he says! He is one of the most insightful and brilliant ministers on the Bible, and the direction our country is going as it relates to our Bible.

You will note the Bible does not even mention America, which gives us cause for some consternation. Does this mean we will become insignificant as a nation by the end time? Listen to Dr. Jeremiah. You will find him extremely enlightening.

Interestingly, it turns out that Ardith lives only half an hour away from Dr. Jeremiah's Shadow Mountain Church in El Cajon, California. Is this a coincidence? I think not.

Don't underestimate the powerful influence of the devil. He is the architect of evil in the world. Pride, hatred, and greed are his weapons. He is the father of lies, the great deceiver, divider, destroyer, and murderer—a sinister mimic, counterfeiter, and impersonator of God. He has his own kingdom, church, gospel, angels, ministers, and hierarchy.

Satan was able to influence an entire nation to support a man with a record of accomplishing absolutely nothing but broken promises and failure, and reject a man like Governor Romney with all kinds of successes as an extraordinary repairman of companies and states. If that's not the devil's work, then what is it?

When I sued the AMA, I could not understand how any organization could stoop so low as to try to create a lie about chiropractic with the intent to destroy its image and ultimately eliminate it, especially when the mastermind of this "containment and elimination" policy had ancestors who went through the same kind of lies and persecution.

Then, I finally came to the realization that we were not fighting the AMA as such, but the devil who got control of key individuals within the AMA and created so much unnecessary pain, suffering, and death.

Satan doesn't need many victims, but just a few victims in the right places.

Dr. John Phillips, prominent pastor, author and public speaker summarized it well when he said:

> *"Our enemies are not people. We must see beyond people. Satan may use people to persecute us, lie to us, cheat us, hurt us, or even kill us. But our real enemy lurks in the shadows of the unseen world, moving people as pawns on the chessboard of time. As long as we see people as enemies and wrestle with them, we will spend our strength in vain."*

I totally concur. We have seen examples of how the devil took over my wife and three daughters, an ordained minister, and his church staff in Park Ridge, a so-called

Christian counselor in Encinitas, California, Ardith's church in Encinitas, California, a judge in Cook Country, Illinois, as well as the other churches in Park Ridge that chose not to be involved.

It's just like my oldest daughter hating me because I added hot water to my wife's restaurant coffee, calling it "controlling and manipulating," or how my middle daughter threw Ardith's and my letters on the ground, then said that she should not have done it but that it was only an impulse, or how my youngest daughter said she hated me and disseminated her hatred in my family for five years, because I did not pay her last two years of college. They are good women, but they are victims and I love them very much and always will. Unfortunately, the devil manipulated them like pawns.

I do NOT suggest that President Obama is deliberately trying to destroy America, nor do I suggest that he is misled by the devil to naively follow his "borrow and spend" mentality to destroy our nation. I do not know what is in his heart. However, if the devil would want to destroy America, then he would do exactly what President Obama is doing. There is no valid evidence showing that Obama's "borrow and spend" policy will ever be effective, but there is ample evidence that it is destructive. This is a given fact. Unless President Obama changes his current approach, he will most certainly, knowingly or unknowingly, destroy America as we know it today. This will be his legacy. I am basically an optimist, but also a realist.

Peter Stoner, Professor Emeritus of Science at Westmont College and author of *Science Speaks,* got together with his cronies, and using the most conservative scientifically-based numbers, concluded that just eight fulfilled predictions with 100 percent accuracy is mathematically established to be one chance in 10 to the 17th power. (That's a one with seventeen zero's) Dr. Stoner sent his figures for review to the committee of the

American Scientific Affiliation, who affirmed them to be dependable and accurate.

To describe the improbability of fulfilling eight of these predictions, it would be like marking a silver dollar, putting it into a pile of silver dollars over nine feet high, covering the entire State of Illinois, and finding that marked coin on the <u>first try</u>. *I fulfilled twenty-three predictions!* This is *Divine Guidance.*

Since the Good Lord does not do things without a reason I believe it was done so that I would write this book revealing my experience and helping others in the process. Hopefully it will help America in its current crisis.

I'm sure some people will scoff at what I say as being absurd, but let them try to explain away how all of these fulfilled predictions, *23 of them, made over 60 years ago, could be anything else but coming from a Higher Power, which is God! If you doubt it and do nothing about it, you will eventually see it for yourself.*

Reflecting back, I have provided solid proof that I was guided and protected by Mrs. Budek, my guardian angel, from a potentially fatal bike accident and from a hold-up at gunpoint by two very dangerous criminals. She cautioned me about a watercraft incident, where I almost drowned. She strongly urged me to change professions, and I ultimately became a chiropractor. She said that I'd meet a doctor who would take a liking to me and become a great help professionally; that I'd write a book, which would become well known and impact a nation. She even predicted that my wife would abandon me and that my daughters would all turn against me, among other events as well. If she was not guiding me, she was cautioning me about impending dangers. She was my guardian angel in the finest sense of the word, and the writing of this book is the ultimate outcome of this book bringing

light into the darkness of ignorance, apathy, indifference, and the intervention of the devil.

* * *

Ending on a lighter note, the Good Lord has used his influence with impressing top politicians who later had a chance to help the chiropractic profession, and I'm sure the Good Lord is working with me on this matter with this book as well. Here are a couple of examples.

President Ronald Regan's first job was working for Dr. B. J. Palmer, who was the President of the Palmer College of Chiropractic and owner of radio station WOC. Regan worked as his sports announcer. His knowledge of chiropractic put him into a position where he could support the value of chiropractic. The call letters WOC were chosen to stand for the "Wonders of Chiropractic."

Senator Hubert Humphrey the 38th Vice President of the United States, sustained a back injury when his model "T" Ford tipped over. He had sought the help of numerous medical specialists, but the only one who could help him was a chiropractor. And so, when Humphrey decided to run for the presidency, he told Dr. Robert Thatcher, who was his chiropractor, that unless he went on the road with him campaigning, that his back could not hold up under the rigorous task of running for president. Dr. Thatcher agreed to travel with him on the road.

Dr. Thatcher enjoyed telling the humorous story about the time he was in Senator Humphrey's hotel room when one of the Secret Servicemen knocked on the door and gave the senator some tranquilizers to help him sleep well that night. He told the Secret Serviceman to lay the napkin down with the pills on the dresser.

After the Secret Serviceman left, Senator Humphrey took the napkin with the pills and said, "Let me take care of this matter." He went into the washroom and "swoosh," the pills went into the toilet. He came out with a towel

115

wrapped around his waist and a big smile on his face and said, "Now, let's get my chiropractic adjustment!"

It is interesting to note that of all things, Senator Humphrey, before he went into politics, was a pharmacist.

It is also ironic to note that had it not been for the pharmacist who discouraged me from fulfilling a prescription for some pills for my back pain, I might not have become a chiropractor.

It has been said that the Lord works in mysterious ways, and Christ certainly proved it to me.

About the Author

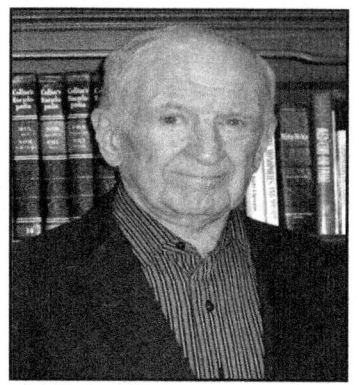 Author Chester A. Wilk, a 1952 graduate of the National College of Chiropractic, is an accomplished professional with a long list of awards and honors for his dedication to the chiropractic profession.

He is known by many in his profession for winning a 14-year long antitrust lawsuit against the American Medical Association to protect the future of chiropractic healthcare.

In 1981, Dr. Wilk was awarded Chiropractor of the Year and noted in *American Chiropractor Magazine*, the largest national chiropractic publication in existence.

He received a Profession Service citation from the American Chiropractic Association, was awarded a Doctor of Humanities degree in 1986 by the Los Angeles College of Chiropractic, and was voted one of the three most respected chiropractors in America.

Additionally, Dr. Wilk received the Janet Travel Annual Award in 2001, which is the highest honor bestowed by the American Academy of Pain Management, a multi-disciplinary pain society, and the largest physician-based society in the U.S.

He also holds an honorary lifetime membership in both the American Chiropractic Association and the International Chiropractor's Association.

In total, Dr. Wilk has received 24 professional awards and has appeared on hundreds of Talk shows.

In addition to his current book, Dr. Wilk has authored seven other books, including *Chiropractic Speaks Out, Chiropractic for Pain, Headaches and Stress, Medicine, Monopolies and Malice,* and *The Case for Christ and Against the Devil.*

To learn more about Dr. Wilk or to contact him, visit one of his websites at: www.chetwilk.com or www.chesterwilk.com.

CPSIA information can be obtained
at www.ICGtesting.com
Printed in the USA
LVOW04s1855040416

482086LV00020B/1042/P

9 781467 557276